PREGNANCY AND INFANTS: MEDICAL, PSYCHOLOGICAL AND SOCIAL ISSUES

MACROSOMIA AND BIRTH WEIGHT

RISK FACTORS, OUTCOMES AND POTENTIAL HEALTH COMPLICATIONS

Pregnancy and Infants: Medical, Psychological and Social Issues

Additional books in this series can be found on Nova's website under the Series tab.

Additional e-books in this series can be found on Nova's website under the e-book tab.

PREGNANCY AND INFANTS: MEDICAL, PSYCHOLOGICAL AND SOCIAL ISSUES

MACROSOMIA AND BIRTH WEIGHT

RISK FACTORS, OUTCOMES AND POTENTIAL HEALTH COMPLICATIONS

LARRY P. HARRIS
EDITOR

NOVA BIOMEDICAL

New York

Library of Congress Cataloging-in-Publication Data

ISBN: 978-1-63483-124-6
Library of Congress Control Number: 2015942061

Published by Nova Science Publishers, Inc. † New York

Contents

Preface

Macrosomia is a term used to describe a neonate with excessive birth weight and is diagnosed when the birth weight exceeds a threshold. Macrosomia is associated with numerous maternal as well as neonatal complications and is, therefore, a major cause of adverse pregnancy outcomes. This book addresses several risk factors, outcomes and potential health complications that may be caused by macrosomia.

Chapter I – Fetal macrosomia is associated with grave maternal and perinatal outcomes. It is associated with increased risk of stillbirth, shoulder dystocia, neonatal hypoglycaemia, hyperbilirubinaemia and hypertrophic cardiomyopathy. Long-term studies have demonstrated that macrosomic offspring have an increased risk of obesity, insulin resistance, type 2 diabetes and cardiovascular disease in later life. For women with pregestational diabetes, the risk of an infant being macrosomic remains extremely high with approximately 50% pregnancies affected. Furthermore, recent national studies suggested the incidence has not fallen over the last twenty years, and has possibly increased in women with pregestational type 1 diabetes. Pedersen's theory of maternal hyperglycaemia leading to fetal hyperglycaemia and subsequent fetal hyperinsulinaemia and fetal overgrowth has been well recognised for fifty years. However, it is important to review recent studies to understand the relationship between blood glucose control during different stages of the pregnancy and infant weight and also maternal diurnal glucose variation and macrosomia. There is an urgent need to establish whether recent studies suggest there is a target maternal glycaemic level at which risk of macrosomia can be reduced. Novel technologies including continuous glucose sensor systems and insulin pumps may hold the key to improved glycaemic control without increased risk of maternal hypoglycaemia. A review of the effectiveness of these newer technologies in reducing macrosomia is essential – both to know their place and also how best to use them to maximise any beneficial effect. It is important to examine macrosomia in type 2 diabetes compared to type 1 diabetes. Despite increased age, obesity and social disadvantage, most studies in women with type 2 diabetes have shown they have better glycaemic control. However, studies of risk of macrosomia in women with type 1 or type 2 diabetes are conflicting with some showing the same and others a lower incidence of macrosomia. The rising obesity epidemic may in part account for the increasing incidence of fetal macrosomia, despite improvements in care. Certainly, gestational weight gain in mothers with type 1 diabetes is a risk factor for macrosomia, independent of glycaemic control or pre-pregnancy BMI.

Chapter II – Although the concurrence of macrosomia and ambiguous genitalia has been described as early as in the Roman Era (as documented by historian accounts of Titus Livius), such an association remains extremely rare. No obvious correlation between these entities has ever been suggested; still, their non-coincidental contingency sheds light on their intermeshing pathophysiological pathways. Ambiguous genitalia are a surrogate of disorders of sex development (DSD) owing to disorders of gonadal development, inadequate biosynthesis or defective action of sex steroids. Macrosomia is a rather frequent disorder, affecting 1-10% of newborns. Elucidating the variants of birth weight, it has been shown that growth hormone (GH)-related parameters are responsible for up to 40% of the variance of birth weight. Fetal overgrowth syndromes encompassing sexual ambiguity include Beckwith-Wiedemann and Simpson-Golabi-Behmel syndromes, in which distinct phenotypic features are prominently exhibited. Another major growth factor implicated in embryonic development is glucocorticoids. Cortisol overproduction could be a possible causative factor of macrosomia via hyperinsulinemia, which is a major determinant of IGF-I levels. A single defect leading to inappropriate activation of the hypothalamic-pituitary-adrenal (HPA) axis, resulting in cortisol and androgen overproduction could be a possible culprit for the concurrent presence of macrosomia and DSD. Besides, Wilms Tumor 1 (WT1) gene encodes a transcription factor acting as a tumor suppressor protein, while it is implicated in the development of both kidney and early gonad in males. Mutant WT1 protein variants have been shown to inadequately suppress IGF-I receptor promoter activity. Consequently, macrosomia and ambiguous genitalia may be concomitant findings in WT1 related disorders. The aim of the present review is to explore the possible pathophysiological mechanisms whose interplay could result in the co-existence of macrosomia and ambiguous genitalia in neonates.

Chapter III – Infant birth weight is known to be dependent on the interplay of nature and nurture. An excessive birth weight has been associated with definite socio-biological maternal characteristics which in part contribute to the genetic makeup of the child and to determining the degree of nutritional capacity made available to the child during intrauterine existence. Macrosomic infants are more likely to be born to relatively older multiparous mothers who are obese and potentially diabetic exhibiting excessive weight gain during pregnancy – all features promoting abundant nutrient availability during intrauterine life. The excessive birth weight of the infant further poses increased perinatal risks to both the mother and child increasing the likelihood for intrapartum problems including prolonged labour and foetal anoxia, an increased risk for operative delivery with the related maternal and infant morbidity, and risks for shoulder dystocia. Besides the short-term problems to the infant posed by the prolonged labour and intrapartum trauma, macrosomia is also associated with long-term metabolic consequences for the child with a greater predisposition to childhood adiposity and adulthood carbohydrate intolerance.

Chapter IV – Objective: The effect of cigarette smoking on the ratio of Placenta Weight vs Birth Weight (PW/BW) is influenced by many factors. The authors have compared the effect of cigarette smoking on BW and PW in two Italian populations living in different environments. Methods: The authors have studied 384 newborn infants from the White population of Rome and 404 newborn infants from the population of Penne. In the metropolitan area of Rome the environmental pollution is high while the rural population of Penne lives in a pure environment. Results: The negative effect of smoking on BW is much stronger in Rome than in Penne. No effect on PW is present in Penne and only a slight not statistically significant effect in Rome. In young women there is a less marked effect of smoking on BW. No differences is observed between sexes. Conclusion: Besides confirming previous observations on the greater effect of maternal smoking on BW as compared to PW, the data suggest that environmental pollution may enhance the effect of smoking. A cumulative action of toxic substances of cigarette smoking on the reproductive apparatus may result in a more evident effect of smoking on intrauterine development in older women.

In: Macrosomia and Birth Weight
Editor: Larry P. Harris

ISBN: 978-1-63483-124-6

Chapter I

Macrosomia in Offspring of Women with Pregestational Type 1 and Type 2 Diabetes: Identifying Risk Factors to Improve Outcomes

Dr. Alice Hurrell and Dr. Rosemary Temple
[1]Speciality Registrar in Obstetrics and Gynaecology
Whipps Cross University Hospital
Leytonstone, London, UK
[2]Consultant Physician in Diabetes and Endocrinology
Norfolk and Norwich University Hospital NHS Trust,
Colney Lane, Norwich, UK

Abstract

Fetal macrosomia is associated with grave maternal and perinatal outcomes. It is associated with increased risk of stillbirth, shoulder dystocia, neonatal hypoglycaemia, hyperbilirubinaemia and hypertrophic cardiomyopathy. Long-term studies have demonstrated that macrosomic offspring have an increased risk of obesity, insulin resistance, type 2 diabetes and cardiovascular disease in later life. For women with pregestational diabetes, the risk of an infant being macrosomic remains extremely high with approximately 50% pregnancies affected. Furthermore, recent national studies suggested the incidence has not fallen over the last twenty years, and has possibly increased in women with pregestational type 1 diabetes.

Pedersen's theory of maternal hyperglycaemia leading to fetal hyperglycaemia and subsequent fetal hyperinsulinaemia and fetal overgrowth has been well recognised for fifty years. However, it is important to review recent studies to understand the relationship between blood glucose control during different stages of the pregnancy and infant weight and also maternal diurnal glucose variation and macrosomia. There is an urgent need to establish whether recent studies suggest there is a target maternal glycaemic level at which risk of macrosomia can be reduced.

Novel technologies including continuous glucose sensor systems and insulin pumps may hold the key to improved glycaemic control without increased risk of maternal hypoglycaemia. A review of the effectiveness of these newer technologies in reducing macrosomia is essential – both to know their place and also how best to use them to maximise any beneficial effect.

It is important to examine macrosomia in type 2 diabetes compared to type 1 diabetes. Despite increased age, obesity and social disadvantage, most studies in women with type 2 diabetes have shown they have better glycaemic control. However, studies of risk of macrosomia in women with type 1 or type 2 diabetes are conflicting with some showing the same and others a lower incidence of macrosomia. The rising obesity epidemic may in part account for the increasing incidence of fetal macrosomia, despite improvements in care. Certainly, gestational weight gain in mothers with type 1 diabetes is a risk factor for macrosomia, independent of glycaemic control or pre-pregnancy BMI.

Introduction

Fetal macrosomia is a significant problem in women with pregestational diabetes. In 1989 the St Vincent declaration set out goals to achieve pregnancy outcomes in women with diabetes the same as those in women without diabetes (Colstrup et al., 2013). Despite efforts to achieve this, the incidence of fetal macrosomia remains dramatically increased and is the most common complication of pregnancy for women with pregestational diabetes (MacIntosh et al., 2006). Fifty years ago, Pedersen hypothesised that maternal hyperglycaemia led to fetal hyperglycaemia, subsequent fetal hyperinsulinaemia and ultimately fetal overgrowth. This is still thought to be the likely underlying aetiology of fetal macrosomia in pregestational diabetes. However, despite the long-standing recognition of this theory, attempts to reduce this common complication have failed.

Defining the Problem of Macrosomia

Healthcare professionals are challenged by the widely varying definition of fetal macrosomia and this has hampered efforts to truly define and drive down the incidence (Sacks, 2010). Terms such as 'macrosomia' and 'large-for-gestational-age' (LGA) may be used interchangeably, although they refer to slightly distinct phenomena. Macrosomia has often been defined in terms of absolute birth weight, and may be described as a birth weight greater than 4000 or 4500 grams (Sacks 2010, Modanlou et al., 1980). However, this fails to take into account confounding by gestational age. By contrast, a baby who is large-for-gestational-age describes an infant who is above the 90th centile, when considering the influence of gestational age and gender, although not ethnicity (Sacks 2010, Murphy et al., 2011). However, this requires customised growth charts, adjusted for gestational age and gender. In a small number of studies, extreme-large-for-gestational-age (extreme-LGA) refers to infants above the 97.5th centile. Unfortunately, in some of these studies, infants are described as being large-for-gestational age, with no immediately apparent distinction. It is worthy of note that neither of these terms considers whether body composition is appropriate and we are still striving for better measures of disproportionate body composition (Persson et al., 2012).

Most recent studies of pregnancy outcomes in women with diabetes have overcome this difficulty by defining macrosomia as large-for-gestational-age (LGA) in their methods. Unless otherwise specified, when referring to macrosomia in this chapter, this is defined as an infant above the 90th growth centile, matched for gestational age and gender.

Prevalence of Macrosomia in Pregestational Diabetes

Several large and longitudinal population-based studies have shown that, despite best efforts to improve antenatal care for women with diabetes and particularly glycaemic control, the incidence of LGA is rising. This is in contrast to some studies showing a reduction in the incidence of macrosomia in gestational diabetes mellitus (Vaarasmaki et al., 2001). The underlying cause of this worrying trend needs to be carefully examined, as the rate of macrosomia appears to be increasing despite apparently good glycaemic control and whilst the rate of other adverse outcomes, such as major malformations and stillbirth, is declining (Persson et al., 2011).

A large systematic review of national studies of outcomes of pregnancies in women with pregestational type 1 diabetes found an overall macrosomia rate of 54.2%, compared with 10% in non-diabetic pregnancies (Colstrup et al., 2013). Similar rates of macrosomia have been seen all across Europe, for instance in Holland, Denmark, Sweden, the United Kingdom and Ireland (see Table 1).

Table 1. A table to demonstrate the incidence of LGA / Macrosomia in Type 1 Diabetes. Numbers expressed as percentage of population

Incidence of LGA (defined as birth weight >90th centile) in Type 1 Diabetes				
Author	*Year*	*Location*	*Type 1 Diabetes*	*Control Population*
Penney	2003	Scotland	55.0	
Evers	2004	Netherlands	45.1	10.0
Jensen	2004	Denmark	62.5	
Holman	2011	East Anglia	45.2	
Persson	2011	Sweden	47.3	9.9
Al-Agha	2012	Ireland	29.0	16.0
Colstrup	2013	Systematic Review	54.2	10.0
Incidence of Extreme-LGA (defined as birth weight >97.7th centile) in Type 1 Diabetes				
Author	*Year*		*Type 1 Diabetes*	*Control Population*
Evers	2004	Netherlands	24.1	
Vaarasmaki	2001	Finland	34.7	3.2
Persson	2009	Sweden	35.0	3.8
Klemetti	2012	Finland	32 - 40	
Incidence of Macrosomia (defined as birth weight >4000g) in Type 1 Diabetes				
Author	*Year*		*Type 1 Diabetes*	*Control Population*
Evers	2004	Netherlands	23.8	
Glinianaia	2012	North England	50.4	
Incidence of Severe Macrosomia (defined as birth weight >4500g) in Type 1 Diabetes				
Author	*Year*	*Location*	*Type 1 Diabetes*	*Control Population*
Evers	2004	Netherlands	7.1	
Jensen	2004	Denmark	8.0	3.4

In Sweden, the incidence of extreme-LGA is increasing, with a rate of 35.0% in 1998 – 2003, compared to 27.6% in 1991 – 1997 (Persson et al., 2009). When compared to the rate in the same population from 1982 – 1985, the results are even more striking, with an absolute increase of 11% and a relative increase of approximately 50% (Persson et al. 2009, Hanson et al., 1993). In contrast, the rate of extreme-LGA in the general population only increased from 3.4 – 3.8%. During the overall study period, the authors found a significant increase in the level of obesity, both in women with diabetes and the background population (Persson et al., 2009) and this may go some way towards explaining the rising incidence of extreme LGA.

Risk Factors for Macrosomia

Risk factors for macrosomia in pregestational diabetes include maternal age, ethnicity, multi-parity, fetal gender, glycaemic control, pre-pregnancy BMI and gestational weight gain. Given that several of these variables are non-modifiable, we will focus on glycaemic control and the influence of maternal obesity and gestational weight gain.

Glycaemic Control

The relationship between hyperglycaemia and fetal growth has been long established. However, it has also been observed that macrosomia can occur in a pregnancy where there has been seemingly good glycaemic control (Cohen et al., 2008). As glucose control is potentially one of the most modifiable risk factors related to macrosomia, it is essential to examine this relationship very closely. As we are focusing on macrosomia in pregestational diabetes, we have excluded studies in women with gestational diabetes.

Overall Glycaemic Control

Over the last twenty years, a number of studies in women with type 1 diabetes have used glycosylated haemoglobin (HbA1c) as a measure of overall glycaemic control and have established a clear relationship between higher HbA1c levels and fetal macrosomia (Wyse et al. 1994, Evers et al. 2004, Glinianaia et al., 2012). Other studies have used different measures of maternal blood glucose monitoring including self-recorded glucose values, downloaded measurements and continuous glucose monitoring and have confirmed the relationship between hyperglycaemia and macrosomia (Sturrock et al. 2001, Mello et al. 2000, Kerssen et al., 2007). However, repeated observations using glycosylated haemoglobin have demonstrated that this relationship then appears to reverse, whereby extremely poor glycaemic control is associated with growth retardation (Rackham et al., 2009).

A recent large study of women with type 1 diabetes has improved our understanding in this area by defining risk of macrosomia at different glycosylated haemoglobin levels (Maresh et al., 2015). In this study, pregnancy outcomes were assessed prospectively in 725 women with type 1 diabetes who had participated in the diabetes and pre-eclampsia intervention trial. HbA1c was measured at 26 weeks gestation (576 women) and 34 weeks gestation (505 women) and the relationship with incidence of macrosomia was explored. HbA1c below 42mmol/mol was used as the reference value. The authors found that even a modest elevation of HbA1c of 42 to 47mmol/mol at 26 weeks gestation was associated with an increased risk of large-for-gestational-age (odds ratio 1.7, 95% confidence interval 1.0 – 3.0). This risk increased progressively with increasing HbA1c, with an odds ratio of 2.5 at 48 – 52mmol/mol, 3.2 at 53 – 58mmol/mol and 3.7 at greater than 59mmol/mol. Results were similar at 34 weeks gestation, with an odds ratio of 1.9 with an HbA1c of 42 – 47mmol/mol, rising to 5.6 with an HbA1c of 53 – 58mmol/mol. Interestingly, the odds ratio then decreased to 2.9 with an HbA1c greater than 59mmol/mol, possibly due to a greater proportion of growth restricted infants exposed to severe hyperglycaemia. All odds ratios were adjusted for maternal age, BMI, social class, ethnicity, parity, smoking status and duration of diagnosis of diabetes. This study highlights how risk of macrosomia is increased with relatively mild hyperglycaemia.

Early or Late Glycaemic Control – Which Matters Most?

Although early studies suggested early glycaemic control may be an important contributor to risk of macrosomia, more recent studies have generally established a relationship between late glycaemic control and macrosomia.

Evidence Against Early Glycaemic Control

Examining the relationship between preconception care (PCC) and macrosomia is important to understand whether there is any relationship between early glycaemia and macrosomia. PCC studies in women with type 1 diabetes have consistently shown an association between PCC and improved glycaemic control in the first trimester. A study of PCC in 680 women with pregestational type 1 or type 2 diabetes found no relationship between preconception care and risk of macrosomia (Murphy et al., 2010).

Furthermore, a recent systematic review examined the relationship between PCC and pregnancy outcomes (Wahabi et al., 2010). Although there were only a small number of studies on PCC and macrosomia, there was no significant reduction in risk of LGA with PPC. There has therefore been no recent evidence supporting a relationship between glycaemia in the first trimester and macrosomia.

Evidence for Late Glycaemic Control

There have been many studies in recent years, using a variety of measures of maternal glycaemia, which have shown that risk of macrosomia is increased with hyperglycaemia in later pregnancy. Mello and colleagues showed, in women with type 1 diabetes, that risk of macrosomia was increased with poor glycaemic control in the second trimester, even if glycaemic improved in the third trimester (Mello et al., 2000). In a study of 98 women with type 1 diabetes, there were significantly fewer LGA babies in women with a mean blood glucose below 95 mg/dL. A small study using continuous glucose monitoring also demonstrated a relationship between elevated glucose levels in the second trimester and risk of LGA (Kerssen et al., 2007). Finally, the Maresh et al. study has established a clear relationship between second and third trimester hyperglycaemia and risk of macrosomia, with generally increasing risk of macrosomia with increasing HbA1c level (Maresh et al., 2015).

These studies all emphasise the importance of optimisation of later blood glucose levels to reduce risk of macrosomia.

Pre- and Post-prandial Glycaemic Control

The relationship between timing of elevated glucose levels and macrosomia is unclear, with studies producing conflicting results.

Evidence for Post-prandial Hyperglycaemia

The Diabetes in Early Pregnancy Study in 323 women with type 1 diabetes showed that an elevated 1-hour post-prandial glucose level predicted rate of macrosomia but there was no relationship with pre-prandial blood glucose (Jovanovic-Peterson et al., 1991). Furthermore, a study of 111 women with type 1 diabetes found no relationship between fasting glucose and macrosomia but a 1-hour value below 130mg/dl was associated with a reduction of LGA risk (Combs et al., 1992). Finally, a small randomised control trial highlighted the importance of post-prandial glycaemia to improve fetal outcome (Manderson et al., 2003).

Evidence for Fasting / Pre-prandial / Mean Hyperglycaemia

In contrast, a study of 70 women with type 1 diabetes showed a relationship between pre-prandial glucose values and risk of LGA (Aschwald et al., 2009). A further study analysing computerised blood glucose levels throughout pregnancy in 47 women with type 1 diabetes showed a relationship between mean blood glucose values and birth weight (Sturrock et al., 2001). Furthermore, the aforementioned study by Maresh et al. in 2015 found that significant trends were demonstrated with large-for-gestational age with pre-prandial glycaemia at both 26 and 34 weeks gestation.

In conclusion, hyperglycaemia in the second half of pregnancy is an important predictor of macrosomia. We have established a clear target for glycosylated haemoglobin to reduce risk. However, to date, it is not completely clear whether we should be focussing on reducing pre-prandial, post-prandial or mean blood glucose levels in order to reduce the burden of macrosomia.

Maternal Obesity

The World Health Organisation has described the dramatically increasing incidence in obesity as a pandemic nutritional disorder (Dixit and Girling,, 2008). A striking 24% of women in the UK are obese, whilst in women aged 35 to 64 years, 32% are overweight and 21% are obese. The prevalence of obesity amongst women booking for antenatal care has been described as 8 – 11%, however other studies have shown up to 20% may be obese (Dixit and Girling,, 2008). Similarly, the prevalence of obesity amongst diabetic mothers is drastically increasing. In a large study from Finland, in 1989 – 1992 the proportions of overweight and obese type 1 diabetic pregnancies were 19.4 and 1.8%, rising to a staggering 32.8 and 9.8% respectively in 2004 – 2008 (Klemetti et al., 2012). It is noteworthy that these results were based on patient-reported pre-pregnancy height and weight. Therefore this may represent an underestimation of the problem.

Obesity has been associated with macrosomia, both in the non-diabetic population, in women with gestational diabetes and in pregestational diabetes (Sebire et al. 2001, Dennedy et al. 1997, Cundy et al. 1993, Klemetti et al., 2012). In a large population-based study in non-diabetic women, the odds ratio for macrosomia (defined as birth weight >4000g) was 1.7 for obese women and 1.9 for morbidly obese women (Weiss et al., 2004). In diabetic pregnancies, numerous studies have demonstrated that pre-pregnancy BMI is an independent risk factor for macrosomia in multiple logistic regression analysis models, although in some studies the reported increased risk was relatively small. One study showed an odds ratio of 1.05 (Klemetti et al., 2012), whilst another showed an odds ratio of 1.6 (Ehrenberg et al. 2004, Cundy et al., 1993). Although the effect may be small, this is a modifiable risk factor and may be an important aspect that may be improved pre-pregnancy.

Gestational Weight Gain

Recommended weight gain during pregnancy is unfortunately a neglected topic and many women are simply not provided with any information (Sacks, 2010). This signifies that an opportunity to change a modifiable risk factor for macrosomia is being missed, as excessive gestational weight gain has been well documented as an independent risk factor for macrosomia (Egan et al., 2014). The Institute of Medicine has issued recommendations for gestational weight gain, such that there should be an inverse relationship between pre-pregnancy BMI and recommended gestational weight gain (Rasmussen et al. 2009, Sacks, 2010). Despite this, studies have shown that 30% of healthcare professionals do not provide any information to patients regarding gestational weight gain, and of those who do give information, only 37 – 49% gave advice within the Institute of Medicine recommendations (Cogswell et al. 1999, Stotland et al., 2005). Furthermore, these studies provide evidence that women may follow the advice they are given – as if women were advised to gain less or more than the recommendations, they generally did gain less or more weight (Sacks, 2010). Finally, restriction of gestational weight gain by diet and exercise has shown an improvement in outcomes in gestational diabetic pregnancies, including the incidence of macrosomia (Crowther et al. 2005, Landon et al., 2009).

Morbidity and Mortality Secondary to Macrosomia

Maternal Consequences of Macrosomia

Diabetes (in the absence of macrosomia) increases the risk of shoulder dystocia by approximately two- to four-fold, compared to infants of the same weight of non-diabetic mothers (Acker et al. 1985, Nesbitt et al., 1998). However, macrosomic offspring of diabetic mothers are particularly at risk. One recent study showed a rate of shoulder dystocia of 27.4% for LGA infants, compared to 4.7% for normally grown infants, with an almost 6-fold increased risk (RR 5.8, Evers et al., 2004). This same study showed a neonatal morbidity rate of over 80%, where neonatal morbidity was defined as one or more neonatal complication. A longitudinal study looking at the rate of shoulder dystocia over 24 years found an odds ratio of 3.8 for pregestational diabetes, and 5.1 for fetal macrosomia (Dandolu et al., 2005). During the study period, there has been a 10-fold increase in the rate of shoulder dystocia, from 0.2% in 1979 to 2.1% in 2003. This may reflect the rising incidence of macrosomia, in addition to increasing levels of obesity, excessive gestational weight gain, gestational diabetes and pregestational diabetes.

The propensity towards shoulder dystocia amongst infants of diabetic mothers is likely due to excessive fat deposition in the upper body, resulting from fetal hyperinsulinaemia. One study found that for every 250g increment of birth weight above 3750g, infants of diabetic women were more likely to encounter a shoulder dystocia than the same size infants of non-diabetic women (Langer et al., 2001).

Shoulder dystocia may result in grave consequences for mother and baby. Maternal morbidity includes post-partum haemorrhage (11%) and perineal trauma, with approximately 4% sustaining a third or fourth degree tear (RCOG Green-top Guideline No. 42 on Shoulder Dystocia,, 2012). Infants are at risk of hypoxic-ischaemic brain injury and brachial plexus injuries, which occur in 2 to 16% of cases. Furthermore, larger babies may be more likely to sustain permanent neurological damage. The CEMACH study of 3733 mothers with pregestational diabetes found a ten-fold increase in the incidence of Erb's palsy in infants of diabetic mothers, compared to an incidence of 0.45 per 1000 births in the general population. Unlike in non-diabetic mothers, elective Caesarean section is therefore recommended in pregestational diabetes if the estimated fetal weight is >4500g. One would hope that by minimising incidence of macrosomia, a significant proportion of shoulder dystocia may be prevented.

Furthermore, macrosomia is associated with other complications of labour, including perinatal hypoxic-ischaemia, obstructed labour, instrumental delivery and emergency Caesarean section, with associated increased maternal morbidity (Weindling 2009, Hawdon, 2011).

Fetal Consequences of Macrosomia

Stillbirth

Most worrying of the complications resulting from macrosomia is the increased risk of unexplained stillbirth (Evers et al., 2002). The UK 2002 – 2003 CEMACH study demonstrated that women with pre-existing diabetes are five times more likely to suffer a stillbirth, and this is closely linked to glycaemic control, particularly suboptimal third trimester HbA1c (CEMACH, 2005)). Other national studies have also shown very elevated stillbirth rates in women with type 1 diabetes (Evers et al. 2004, Lauenborg et al., 2003).

There is a curvilinear relationship between HbA1c and birth weight amongst perinatal deaths, such that a low HbA1c is associated with normal birth weight, moderately increased HbA1c results in increased birth weight and significantly raised HbA1c causes fetal growth restriction (Rackham et al., 2009). This is likely to be explained by the Pedersen hypothesis, which states that maternal hyperglycaemia is reflected by fetal hyperglycaemia, resulting in fetal hyperinsulinaemia due to pancreatic beta-cell stimulation. Hyperinsulinaemia results in excessive growth, excess subcutaneous fat and hepatic glycogen storage (Mathiesen et al., 2011). This altered fetal metabolism results in relative fetal hypoxia, as demonstrated by the fact that fetal umbilical venous erythropoietin concentration, a marker of hypoxic stress, correlates with third trimester HbA1c (Widness et al., 1990). Furthermore, fetal amniotic fluid insulin levels correlate with umbilical venous erythropoietin levels, independently of maternal HbA1c, which may mean that fetal hyperinsulinaemia causes hypoxia above and beyond the effect of maternal hyperglycaemia (Mathiesen et al., 2011). Fetal hypoxia is clearly linked to stillbirth, as one study showed 64 out of 93 perinatal deaths in type 1 and type 2 diabetic pregnancies were due to antepartum asphyxia (Rackham et al., 2009) and another study found high amniotic fluid erythropoeitin concentrations prior to stillbirth (Teramo et al., 2004). However, despite high levels of fetal surveillance, prediction of stillbirth amongst diabetic patients is poor and emphasis should be placed on new methods for identifying fetuses at risk.

Neonatal Morbidity

Neonatal complications in infants of diabetic pregnancies are particularly prevalent in macrosomic infants, as both are reflections of poor diabetic control. Neonates may be troubled by a stormy postnatal course, including hypoglycaemia, hyperbilirubinaemia, respiratory distress syndrome, admission to the Neonatal Unit (NNU) and, rarely, hypertrophic cardiomyopathy.

It is paramount to monitor for hypoglycaemia resulting from fetal hyperinsulinaemia. However, this may be over-diagnosed and result in unnecessary admission to NNU if blood sugars are checked too soon after delivery, capturing the normal physiological fall in blood glucose, which reaches a nadir at 1-hour post-delivery and stabilises by 3 hours post-natally (Weindling, 2009). Fetal hyperinsulinaemia results in relative cellular hypoxia in-utero, which stimulates fetal erythropoietin production, which in turn increases red cell production. Postnatal red cell lysis then leads to hyperbilirubinaemia and jaundice, sometimes necessitating exchange transfusion (Hawdon, 2011). Infants of diabetic mothers are at increased risk of respiratory distress as high glucose levels impacts surfactant synthesis and secretion and there may be fewer type II alveolar pneumocytes (Weindling, 2009). In a historic UK survey of pregestational diabetes, there were fortunately no cases of hypertrophic cardiomyopathy (Miller et al., 1943). However, some studies have shown that hyperinsulinaemia causes excessive septal growth and in one study of 12 infants with cardiac hypertrophy, 10 out of 12 were macrosomic (Halliday, 1981). In the largest prenatal study of cardiomyopathy, 75% of 64 fetuses had ventricular septal hypertrophy on fetal echo (Veille et al., 1992).

Despite all these concerning complications, neonates may be unnecessarily subjected to admission to SCBU. This maternal separation may negatively impact bonding and breast-feeding, additionally contributing to post-natal depression. In the CEMACH survey of 3733 women with pregestational diabetes, 56% of neonates were admitted to NNU, compared to 10% in the general population. Furthermore, 33% of term infants were admitted to NNU, compared to 10% in the general population, and a worrying 67% of these were assessed as avoidable (Hawdon, 2010). Therefore, it is paramount that appropriate and specialist planning of neonatal management takes place in advance of delivery, to optimise care and prevent unnecessary or routine NNU admission, based on historical policies.

Long-term Consequences of Macrosomia

It is increasingly recognised that exposure to a diabetic metabolic milieu in-utero may have implications that persist far beyond the neonatal period. Macrosomic infants may in later life be troubled by obesity, metabolic syndrome, impaired glucose tolerance, diabetes and increased cardiovascular risk (Fraser et al. 2014, Glinianaia et al. 2012, Persson et al. 2011, Rijpert et al., 2009). A systematic review of nine studies investigating BMI in offspring of diabetic pregnancies concluded that maternal diabetes predisposed offspring to a significantly increased BMI (Philipps et al., 2011). However, this association was attenuated when they only included the three studies that adjusted for maternal BMI. Compelling evidence comes from sibling studies comparing offspring before and after maternal diagnosis of diabetes; one study found mean BMI was 2.6 kg/m2 higher and the odds ratio for offspring diagnosis of diabetes was 3.7 (Lawler et al. 2011, Dabelea et al., 2000).

Neonatal macrosomia has been found to be an independent risk factor for adult metabolic syndrome in animal studies (Hermann et al., 2010). A human study found that the combination of LGA and gestational diabetes resulted in a greater prevalence of metabolic syndrome and an increased odds ratio for insulin resistance of 10.4, when compared to LGA without diabetes and appropriately grown infants (Boney et al., 2005). Unfortunately, there is limited data specifically comparing long-term outcomes of macrosomic offspring compared to normally grown offspring of mothers with pregestational diabetes. One small study of 51 infants of diabetic mothers showed that macrosomia significantly increased the risk of impaired glucose tolerance in 2 – 5 year olds (Buinauskiene et al., 2004). A meta-analysis showed that increased birth weight increased the probability of developing childhood type 1 diabetes, independently of maternal diabetes, such that an increase in birth weight by 500g resulted in a 3% increased risk (Cardwell et al., 2010).

Can New Technologies Reduce Risk of Macrosomia?

In the past two decades, there have been huge technological advances to aid patients with type 1 diabetes to optimise their blood glucose control. These advances have included continuous subcutaneous insulin infusion (CSII) or insulin pumps to improve insulin delivery and continuous glucose monitoring (CGM) so blood glucose can be monitored throughout the day and night. These tools are increasingly used by people living with diabetes and there is now considerable research showing how they can improve glycaemic control while reducing risk of hypoglycaemia. In contrast, research in relation to their use during pregnancy and maternal and fetal outcomes remains limited.

Continuous Glucose Monitoring

The development of CGM over the last decade has led to a much greater understanding both of what are physiological glucose levels during pregnancy in women without diabetes and also the erratic and often very high blood glucose levels that can be seen in women during pregnancy who appear to be well controlled (as judged by their glycosylated haemoglobin levels). CGM systems measure glucose levels in the interstitial fluid every ten seconds, providing an average interstitial glucose value every five minutes (288 values a day). These small, disposable glucose sensing devices are easy to wear and can now be worn for seven days. Recently developed real-time CGM systems display continuous glucose values and have alarm functions to warn about impending hypo- or hyperglycaemia.

To date, there are two published randomised controlled studies of CGM use in pregnancy. In the first, a two centre study from the UK, women were randomised to wearing CGM every four to six weeks throughout pregnancy or to routine care with no CGM (Murphy et al., 2008). 71 women participated in the study, 46 with type 1 diabetes and 25 with type 2 diabetes. Glycosylated haemoglobin was significantly lower in the intervention group at 32-36 weeks gestation (5.8% vs 6.4%, p = 0.007). Compared with infants of mothers in the control arm, those of mothers in the intervention arm had a reduced risk of macrosomia (odds ratio 0.36, 95% confidence interval 0.13 to 0.98, p = 0.05). These results confirmed CGM use improved glycaemia control and reduced risk of macrosomia.

Another recent RCT by. investigated the effect of intermittent real time CGM use during pregnancy on pregnancy outcome in 154 women with pre-existing diabetes (123 with type 1 diabetes and 31 with type 2 diabetes) (Secher et al., 2013). The rate of macrosomia was not significantly different between the intervention group (43%) and the control group (30%) (p = 0.09). Also, HbA1c levels were similar in both groups. The investigators concluded that intermittent CGMS use did not improve glycaemic control in pregnancy nor did it improve pregnancy outcome. However there were a number of limitations to this study. These included limited sensor use (only 64% women used CGM as per study protocol and the focus of the study to reduce hypoglycaemia (alarms were activated for hypoglycaemia interrupting sleep in a third of CGM users).

Clearly, more data are required before routine clinical use of CGM in pregnancy can be fully endorsed. An international Continuous Glucose Monitoring in Women with Type 1 Diabetes in Pregnancy Trial (CONCEPTT) is now underway and will evaluate the role of continuous real-time CGM before (ie during preconception care) and during pregnancy. Ultimately, it may be it is not the devices per se but how patients, their spouses/significant others, and health professionals interact with CGM that will determine outcomes.

Continuous Subcutaneous Insulin Infusion

Pump therapy or CSII is much more able to closely mimic physiological insulin secretion and has many advantages over the tradition basal/ bolus insulin regimes. These include improved glycaemic control (as reflected by glycosylated haemoglobin), reductions in severe hypoglycaemic episodes, reductions in total daily insulin requirements and improved quality of life (due to reduced fear of hypoglycaemia and improved lifestyle). It would therefore seem logical that CSII may be associated with improved pregnancy outcomes.

CSII is now being used with increasing frequency during pregnancy in women with type 1 diabetes.

However, robust clinical evidence, in the form of randomised controlled studies, remains small. A systematic review, comparing CSII to multiple daily injections (MDI,) included only two RCTs (61 pregnancies) (Farrar et al., 2007). They found no significant difference between groups in maternal hyper- or hypoglycaemia or in rate of fetal macrosomia (defined as birth weight greater than 4000g).

There have been many small retrospective studies comparing maternal and fetal outcomes in women using CSII or MDI during pregnancy (Mello et al. 2015, Neff et al. 2014, Chico et al. 2010, Brottomesso et al., 2011). The more recent studies are shown in Table 2.

These studies consistently show reduced daily insulin requirements in women using CSII. Unfortunately, the small numbers in the studies combined with the lack of correction for potential confounders (such as parity or maternal weight), means that we still lack robust data to recommend use of CSII either to improve maternal glycaemia or to prevent macrosomia. There is an urgent need to have a large randomised controlled study of CSII use versus MDI in pregnancy. However, with the rapid advances in new technologies, it may seem prudent to do such a study using sensor-augmented pumps.

Table 2. Recent retrospective studies comparing CSII use with MDI

First author	Number of women (number using CSII)	Effect on maternal HbA1c (in CSII group)	Macrosomia (in CSII group)
Mello	53 (35)	No difference	No difference
Wender-Ozegowska	128 (64)	Reduced hypoglycaemia	No difference
Chico	315 (103)	No difference	Increased risk
Brutomesso	144 (100)	Reduced late HbA1c	No difference
Neff	464 (40)	No difference	No difference

Type 2 Diabetes and Macrosomia

With the rapid rise in obesity worldwide, there are increasing numbers of women with type 2 diabetes of reproductive age. Consequently, in recent years, there have been several studies comparing rates of macrosomia in women with type 1 or type 2 diabetes. Earlier studies suggested similar rates of macrosomia irrespective of type of diabetes (Balsells et al., 2009). An early study from the East of England (1999-2004) showed similar rates of macrosomia in type 2 and type 1 diabetes (46.5% vs 46.9%) (Roland et al.,

2005). In contrast, a later study (2006-2009) from the same ten hospitals, which included 682 women with type 1 or type 2 diabetes, showed much lower rates of macrosomia (Murphy et al., 2010). These ten hospitals, having recognized the poor outcomes in women with type 2 diabetes during the first study, placed much attention on optimizing glycaemic control throughout pregnancy in women with type 2 diabetes.

Recent studies comparing pregnancies in women with type 1 and type 2 diabetes have identified that women with type 2 diabetes are likely to have a higher pre-pregnancy BMI, be older, more parous and be from a lower socio-economic class. However, they usually enter pregnancy with better glycaemic control than women with type 1 diabetes and have better glycaemia in later pregnancy (Murphy et al., 2011).

Since women with type 2 diabetes have multiple risk factors for macrosomia, it is essential to try to understand which are the more important factors. In the second study from the East of England, including 682 women (40.2% with type 2 diabetes), logistic regression analyses were performed. Across the whole study population, the only significant risk factors for LGA were 3rd trimester HbA1c (OR 1.35) and social disadvantage (OR 0.80) (Murphy et al., 2011). When focusing on women with type 2 diabetes alone, social disadvantage remained a risk factor (OR 0.71) and maternal obesity was also a small risk factor (OR 1.07).

The relationship between social deprivation and risk of macrosomia has not previously been appreciated. We have already presented data suggesting postprandial hyperglycaemia may be an important risk factor for macrosomia. We would therefore speculate that women who are socially disadvantaged may be a eating higher glycaemic index refined carbohydrates which are leading to postprandial hyperglycaemic excursions and subsequent macrosomia.

Defining the Targets

There is now clear data to help us to reduce rates of macrosomia.

Firstly, it is essential to optimize glycaemic control in second and third trimesters of pregnancy.

There is considerable evidence that women should do both pre- and postprandial glucose monitoring. Current international targets are similar between countries and are shown in Table 3 Recent data suggests that we should monitor HbA1c at regular intervals and aim for an HbA1c below 42 mmol/mol, if possible. This should be easily achievable in most women with type 2 diabetes as hypoglycaemia is rarely a major problem. However, in women with type 1 diabetes, this may not be achievable without significant hypoglycaemia, even if using insulin pumps and CGMS. If women have an HbA1c above 42 mmol/mol, close obstetric surveillance is essential, as the risk of macrosomia and associated problems will be two to five times higher. Women should be advised of these risks.

At present, there is reasonable agreement between different countries over glucose targets throughout pregnancy (Table 3). However, Hernandez and colleagues recently pooled results of studies of glucose levels in women without diabetes during pregnancy, and found much lower mean blood glucose levels than previously thought (fasting plasma glucose 71.8 mg/dL, 1 hour postprandial glucose 109 mg/dL and 2 hour postprandial 99mg/dL0 (Hernandez, 2015). They have suggested that current international glucose targets for women with diabetes may be too high, accounting for our lack of reduction of macrosomia in recent years. Clearer guidance on achieving optimum pre-pregnancy weight and an increased understanding and guidance on gestational weight gain are other important aspects if we are to reduce risk of macrosomia.

Table 3. Comparison of blood glucose targets (expressed in mg/dL) in different countries for women with pregestational diabetes (Hernandez, 2015)

	Fasting	1 hour peak	2 hour peak
American Diabetes Association	<90	100-129	No target
Endocrine Society	<90	<140	<120
Canadian Diabetes Association	<95	<140	<120
National Institute for Clinical Excellence (UK)	95	<140	<115

Conclusion

Macrosomia is the most common complication of a pregnancy in women with pregestational diabetes. It has many consequences both for the mother and the infant. Furthermore, in later years, the child will be at increased risk of chronic health problems including diabetes and obesity.

We have identified clear and potentially modifiable risk factors, including maternal glycaemia in later pregnancy, maternal pre-pregnancy weight and gestational weight gain. It is now essential that we educate and support women to achieve targets in these areas and optimize health for both the mother and baby.

References

Acker DB; Sachs BP; Friedman EA. Risk factors for shoulder dystocia. *Obstet Gynecol* 1985;66: 762-8.

Al-Agha R; Firth RG; Byrne M; Murray S; Daly S; Foley M; Smith SC; Kinsley BT. Outcome of pregnancy in type 1 diabetes mellitus (T1DMP): results from combined diabetes-obstetrical clinics in Dublin in three university teaching hospitals (1995-2006). *Ir. J. Med. Sci.* 2012 Mar;181(1): 105-9.

Aschwald CL; Catanzaro RB; Weiss EP; Gavard JA; Steitz KA; Mostello DJ. Large-for-gestational-age infants of type 1 diabetic mothers: an effect of preprandial hyperglycaemia? *Gynecol. Endocrinol.* 2009 Oct;25(10): 653-60.

Balsells M; Garcia-Patterson A; Gich I; Corcoy R. Maternal and fetal outcome in women with type 2 versus type 1 diabetes mellitus: a systematic review and meta-analysis. *J. Clin. Endocrinol. Metab.* 2009 Nov;94(11): 4284-91.

Boney CM; Verma A; Tucker R; Vohr BR. Metabolic syndrome in childhood: association with birth weight, maternal obesity, and gestational diabetes mellitus. *Pediatrics.* 2005 Mar;115(3): e290-6.

Bruttomesso D, Bonomo M, Costa S, Dal POs M, Di Cianni et al. Type 1 diabetes control and pregnancy outcomes in women treated with continuous subcutaneous insulin infusion or with insulin glargine and multiple daily injections of rapid acting insulin analogue. *Diabetes Metab*, 2011. 37(5): 426-31.

Buinauskiene J; Baliutaviciene D; Zalinkevicius R. Glucose tolerance of 2- to 5-yr-old offspring of diabetic mothers. *Pediatr. Diabetes.* 2004 Sep:5(3): 143-6.

Cardwell CR; Stene LC; Joner G; Davis EA; Cinek O *et al.* Birthweight and the risk of childhood-onset type 1 diabetes: a meta-analysis of observational studies using individual patient data. *Diabetologia.* 2010 Apr;53(4): 641-51.

Chico A; Saigi I; Garcia-Patterson A; Santos MD; Adelantado JM; Ginovart G; de Leiva A; Corcoy R. Glycemic control and perinatal outcomes of pregnancies complicated by type 1 diabetes: influence of continuous subcutaneous insulin infusion and lispro insulin. *Diabetes Technol. Ther.* 2010 Dec;12(12): 937-45.

Cogswell ME; Scanlon KS; Fein SB; Schieve LA. Medically advised, mother's personal target, and actual weight gain during pregnancy. *Obstet. Gynecol.* 1999 Oct;94(4): 616-22.

Cohen O; Keidar N; Simchen M; Weisz B; Dolitsky M; Sivan E. Macrosomia in well controlled CSII treated Type 1 diabetic pregnancy. *Gynecol. Endocrinol.* 2008 Nov;24(11): 611-3.

Colstrup M; Mathiesen ER; Damm P; Jensen DM; Ringholm L. Pregnancy in women with type 1 diabetes: have the goals of St Vincent declaration been met concerning foetal and neonatal complications? *J. Matern. Fetal. Neonatal. Med.* 2013 Nov;26(17): 1682-6.

Combs CA; Gunderson E; Kitzmiller JL; Gavin LA; Main EK. Relationship of fetal macrosomia to maternal postprandial glucose control during pregnancy. *Diabetes Care.* 1992 Oct;15(10): 1251-7.

Confidential Enquiry into Maternal and Child Health. Pregnancy in women with type 1 and type 2 diabetes in 2002 – 03, England Wales and Northern Ireland. London CEMACH 2005.

Crowther CA; Hiller JE; Moss JR; McPhee AJ; Jeffries WS; Robinson JS; Australian Carbohydrate Intolerance Study in Pregnant Women (ACHOIS) Trial Group. Effect of treatment of gestational diabetes mellitus on pregnancy outcomes. *N. Engl. J. Med.* 2005 Jun 16;352(24): 2477-86.

Cundy T; Gamble G; Manuel A; Townend K; Roberts A. Determinants of birth-weight in women with established and gestational diabetes. *Aust. N Z J. Obstet. Gynaecol.* 1993 Aug;33(3): 249-54.

Dabelea D; Hanson RL; Lindsay RS; Pettitt DJ; Imperatore G; Gabir MM; Roumain J; Bennett PH; Knowler WC. Intrauterine exposure to diabetes conveys risks for type 2 diabetes and obesity: a study of discordant sibships. *Diabetes.* 2000 Dec;49(12): 2208-11.

Dandolu V; Lawrence L; Gaughan JP; Grotegut C; Harmanli OH, Jaspan D; Hernandez E. Trends in the rate of shoulder dystocia over two decades. *J Matern. Fetal. Neonatal.* Med. 2005 Nov; 18(5): 305-10.

Dennedy MC; Avalos G; O'Reilly MW; O'Sullivan EP; Gaffney G; Dunne F. ATLANTIC-DIP: raised maternal body mass index (BMI) adversely affects maternal and fetal outcomes in glucose-tolerant women according to International Association of Diabetes and Pregnancy Study Groups (IADPSG) criteria. *J Clin Endocrinol Metab.* 2012 Apr;97(4): E608-12

Dixit A; Girling JC. Obesity and pregnancy. J. Obstet. Gynaecol. 2008 Jan;28(1): 14-23.

Egan AM; Dennedy MC; Al-Ramli W; Heerey A; Avalos G; Dunne F. ATLANTIC-DIP: excessive gestational weight gain and pregnancy outcomes in women with gestational or pregestational diabetes mellitus. *J. Clin. Endocrinol. Metab*. 2014 Jan;99(1): 212-9.

Ehrenberg HM; Mercer BM; Catalano PM. The influence of obesity and diabetes on the prevalence of macrosomia. *Am. J. Obstet. Gynecol*. 2004 Sep;191(3): 964-8.

Evers IM; de Valk HW; Mol BW; ter Braak EW; Visser GH. Macrosomia despite good glycaemic control in Type 1 diabetic pregnancy; results of a nationwide study in The Netherlands. *Diabetologia*. 2002 Nov;45(11): 1484-9.

Evers IM; de Valk HW; Visser GH. Risk of complications of pregnancy in women with type 1 diabetes: nationwide prospective study in the Netherlands. *BMJ*. 2004 Apr 17;328(7445):915.

Farrar D; Tuffnell DJ; West J. Continuous subcutaneous insulin infusion versus multiple daily injections of insulin for pregnant women with diabetes. *Cochrane Database Syst. Rev*. 2007 Jul 18;(3): CD005542.

Fraser A, Lawlor DA. Long-term health outcomes in offspring born to women with diabetes in pregnancy. *Curr. Diab. Rep*. 2014;14(5): 489.

Glinianaia SV, Tennant PW, Bilous RW, Rankin J, Bell R. HbA(1c) and birthweight in women with pre-conception type 1 and type 2 diabetes: a population-based cohort study. *Diabetologia*. 2012 Dec;55(12): 3193-203

Halliday HL. Hypertrophic cardiomyopathy in infants of poorly-controlled diabetic mothers. *Arch. Dis. Child* 1981;56: 258-63.

Hanson U; Persson B. Outcome of pregnancies complicated by type 1 insulin-dependent diabetes in Sweden: acute pregnancy complications, neonatal mortality and morbidity. *Am. J. Perinatol*. 1993 Jul;10(4): 330-3.

Hawdon JM. Babies born after diabetes in pregnancy: what are the short- and long-term risks and how can we minimise them? *Best. Pract. Res. Clin. Obstet. Gynaecol*. 2011 Feb;25(1): 91-104.

Hermann GM; Dallas LM; Haskell SE; Roghair RD. Neonatal macrosomia is an independent risk factor for adult metabolic syndrome. *Neonatology*. 2010;98(3): 238-44.

Hernandez TL. Glycemic targets in pregnancies affected by diabetes: historical perspective and future directions. *Curr. Diab. Rep*. 2015 Jan;15(1):565.

Holman N; Lewis-Barned N; Bell R; Stephens H; Modder J; Gardosi J; Dornhorst A; Hillson R; Young B; Murphy HR. NHS Diabetes in

Pregnancy Dataset Development Group. *Diabet. Med.* 2011 Jul;28(7): 797-804.

Jensen DM; Damm P; Moelsted-Pedersen L; Ovesen P; Westergaard JG; Moeller M; Beck-Nielsen H. Outcomes in type 1 diabetic pregnancies: a nationwide, population-based study. *Diabetes Care.* 2004 Dec;27(12): 2819-23.

Jovanovic-Peterson L; Peterson CM; Reed GF; Metzger BE; Mills JL; Knopp RH; Aarons JH. Maternal postprandial glucose levels and infant birth weight: the Diabetes in Early Pregnancy Study. The National Institute of Child Health and Human Development – Diabetes in Early Pregnancy Study. *Am. J. Obstet. Gynecol.* 1991 Jan;164(1 Pt 1): 103-11.

Kerssen A; de Valk HW; Visser GH. Increased second trimester maternal glucose levels are related to extremely large-for-gestational-age infants in women with type 1 diabetes. *Diabetes Care.* 2007 May;30(5): 1069-74.

Klemetti M; Nuutila M; Tikkanen M; Kari MA; Hiilesmaa V; Teramo K. Trends in maternal BMI, glycaemic control and perinatal outcome among type 1 diabetic pregnant women in 1989-2008. *Diabetologia.* 2012 Sep;55(9): 2327-34.

Landon MB; Spong CY; Thom E; Carpenter MW; Ramin SM; Casey B; Wapner RJ; Varner MW; Rouse DJ; Thorp JM Jr; Sciscione A; Catalano P; Harper M; Saade G; Lain KY; Sorokin Y; Peaceman AM; Tolosa JE; Anderson GB; Eunice Kennedy Shriver National Institute of Child Health and Human Development Maternal-Fetal Medicine Units Network. A multicentre, randomized trial of treatment for mild gestational diabetes. N. *Engl. J. Med.* 2009 Oct 1;361(14): 1339-48.

Langer O; Berkus MD; Huff RW; Samueloff A. Shoulder dystocia: should the fetus weighing greater than or equal to 4000 grams be delivered by cesarean section? *Am. J. Obstet. Gynecol.* 1991;165: 831-7.

Lauenborg J; Mathiesen E; Oversen P; Westergaard JG; Ekbom P; Molsted-Pedersen L; Damm P. Audit on stillbirths in women with pregestational type 1 diabetes. *Diabetes Care.* 2003 May;26(5): 1385-9.

Lawlor DA; Lichtenstein P; Langstrom N. Association of maternal diabetes mellitus in pregnancy with offspring adiposity into early adulthood: sibling study in a prospective cohort of 280,866 men from 248,293 families. *Circulation.* 2011 Jan 25;123(3): 258-65.

Macintosh MC, Fleming K, Bailey JA, Doylp P, Modder et al. Perinatl mortality and congenital anomalies in babies of women with type 1 and type diabetes in England, Wales and Northern Ireland; a populationmstudy. *BMJ* 2006: 333 (7560); 177.

Manderson JG; Patterson CC; Hadden DR; Traub AI; Ennis C; McCance DR. Preprandial versus postprandial blood glucose monitoring in type 1 diabetic pregnancy: a randomized controlled clinical trial. *Am. J. Obstet. Gynecol.* 2003 Aug;189(2): 507-12.

Maresh MJ; Holmes VA; Patterson CC; Young IS; Pearson DW; Walker JD, McCance DR. Diabetes and Pre-eclampsia Intervention Trial Study Group. Glycemic targets in the second and third trimester of pregnancy for women with type 1 diabetes. *Diabetes Care.* 2015 Jan;38(1): 34-42.

Mathiesen ER; Ringholm L; Damm P. Stillbirth in diabetic pregnancies. *Best Pract. Res. Clin. OBstet. Gynaecol.* 2011 Feb;25(1): 105-11.

Mello G; Biagioni S; Ottanelli S; Nardini C; Tredici Z; Serena C; Marchi L; Mecacci F. Continuous subcutaneous insulin infusion (CSII) versus multiple daily injections (MDI) of rapid-acting insulin analogues and detemir in type 1 diabetic (T1D) pregnant women. *J. Matern. Fetal. Neonatal. Med.* 2015 Feb;28(3): 276-80.

Mello G; Parretti E; Mecacci F; La Torre P; Cioni R; Cianciulli D; Scarselli G. What degree of maternal metabolic control in women with type 1 diabetes is associated with normal body size and proportions in full-term infants? *Diabetes Care.* 2000 Oct;23(10): 1494-8.

Miller HD; Wilson HM. Macrosomia, cardiac hypertrophy, erythroblastosis, and hyperplasia of the islands of Langerhans in infants of diabetic mothers. *J. Pediatr.* 1943;23: 251-66.

Modanlou HD; Dorchester WL; Thorosian A; Freeman RK. Macrosomia – maternal, fetal, and neonatal implications. *Obstet. Gynecol.* 1980;55 420-4.

Murphy HR, Roland JM, Skinner TC, Simmons D, Gurnell E et al. Effectiveness of a regional prepregnancy care programme in women with type 1 and type 2 diabetes: benefits beyond glycaemic control. *Diabetes Care* 2010. 33(12); 2514-20.

Murphy HR; Rayman G; Lewis K; Kelly S; Johal B; Duffield K; Fowler D; Campbell PJ; Temple RC. Effectiveness of continuous glucose monitoring in pregnant women with diabetes: randomized clinical trial. *BMJ.* 2008 Sep 25;337;a1680.

Murphy HR; Roland JM; Skinner TC; Simmons D; Gurnell E; Morrish NJ; Soo SC; Kelly S; Lim B; Randall J; Thompsett S; Temple RC. Effectiveness of a regional prepregnancy care program in women with type 1 and type 2 diabetes: benefits beyond glycemic control. *Diabetes Care.* 2010 Dec;33(12): 2514-20.

Murphy HR; Steel SA; Roland JM; Morris D; Ball V; Campbell PJ; Temple RC. East Anglia Study Group for Improving Pregnancy Outcomes in Women with Diabetes (EASIPOD). Obstetric and perinatal outcomes in pregnancies complicated by Type 1 and Type 2 diabetes: influences of glycaemic control, obesity and social disadvantage. *Diabet. Med.* 2011 Sep;28(9): 1060-7.

Neff KJ; Forde R; Gavin C; Byrne MM; Firth RG; Daly S; McAuliffe FM; Foley M; Coffey M; Coulter-Smith S; Kinsley BT. Pre-pregnancy care and pregnancy outcomes in type 1 diabetes mellitus: a comparison of continuous subcutaneous insulin infusion and multiple daily injection therapy. *Ir. J. Med. Sci.* 2014 Sep;183(3): 397-403.

Nesbitt TS; Gilbert WM; Herrchen B. Shoulder dystocia and associated risk factors with macrosomic infants born in California. *Am. J. Obstet. Gynecol.* 1998;179: 476-80.

Penney GC; Mair G; Pearson DW. Scottish Diabetes in Pregnancy Group. Outcomes of pregnancies in women with type 1 diabetes in Scotland: a national population-based study. *BJOG.* 2003 Mar;110(3): 315-8.

Persson M; Norman M; Hanson U. Obstetric and perinatal outcomes in type 1 diabetic pregnancies: A large, population-based study. *Diabetes Care.* 2009 Nov;32(11): 2005-9.

Persson M; Pasupathy D; Hanson U; Norman M. Birth size distribution in 3,705 infants born to mothers with type 1 diabetes: a population-based study. *Diabetes Care.* 2011 May;34(5): 1145-9.

Persson M; Pasupathy D; Hanson U; Norman M. Disproportionate body composition and perinatal outcome in large-for-gestational-age infants to mothers with type 1 diabetes. *BJOG.* 2012 Apr;119(5): 565-72.

Philipps LH; Santhakumaran S; Gale C; Prior E; Logan KM; Hyde MJ; Modi N. The diabetic pregnancy and offspring BMI in childhood: a systematic review and meta-analysis. *Diabetologia.* 2011 Aug;54(8): 1957-66.

Rackham O; Paize F; Weindling AM. Cause of death in infants of women with pregestational diabetes mellitus and the relationship with glycaemic control. *Postgrad. Med.* 2009 Jul;121(4): 26-32.

Rasmussen KM; Yaktine AL, editors. Weight gain during pregnancy: re-examining the guidelines. Institute of Medicine (US) and National Research Council (US) Committee to Re-examine IOL Pregnancy Weight Guidelines. National Academies press 2009.

Rijpert M; Evers IM; de Vroede MA; de Valk HW; Heijnen CJ; Visser GH. Risk factors for childhood overweight in offspring of type 1 diabetic women with adequate glycemic control during pregnancy: Nationwide follow-up study in the Netherlands. *Diabetes Care*. 2009 Nov;32(11): 2099-104.

Roland JM; Murphy HR; Ball V; Northcote-Wright J; Temple RC. The pregnancies of women with type 2 diabetes: poor outcomes but opportunities for improvement. *Diabetic Med.* 2005 Dec;22(12): 1774-7

Sacks DA. Big babies in pregnancies complicated by diabetes: Is it all about maternal glucose? *Perinatology* 2010; 4: 30-36.

Sebire NJ; Jolly M; Harris JP; Wadsworth J; Joffe M; Beard RW; Regan L; Robinson S. Maternal obesity and pregnancy outcome: a study of 287,213 pregnancies in London. Int. *J. Obes. Relat. Metab. Disord.* 2001 Aug;25(8): 1175-82.

Secher AL, Ringholm L, Andersen HU, Damm P, Mathiesen ER. The effect of real-time continuous glucose monitoring in pregnant women with diabetes: a randomized controlled trial. *Diabetes Care*. 2013 Jul;36(7): 1877-83.

Shoulder Dystocia. Royal College of Obstetricians and Gynaecologists, Green-top Guideline No. 42, 2nd Edition, March 2012.

Stotland NE; Haas JS; Brawarsky P; Jackson RA; Fuentes-Afflick E; Escobar GJ. Body mass index, provider advice, and target gestational weight gain. *Obstet. Gynecol.* 2005 Mar;105(3): 633-8.

Sturrock ND; Fay TN; Pound N; Kirk BA; Danks LE. Analysis of 44,279 blood glucose estimations in relation to outcomes in 80 pregnant diabetic women. *J. Obstet. Gynaecol.* 2001 May;21(3): 253-7.

Teramo K, Kari MA, ERonen M, Markkanen H, Hiilesmaa V. High amniotic fluid erythropoietin levels are associated with an increased frequency of fetal and neonatal morbidity in type 1 diabetic pregnancies. *Diabetologia.* 2004 Oct;47(10): 1695-703.

Vaarasmaki M; Gissler M; Hartikainen AL. A uniform regimen enables decentralized care of diabetic pregnancies. *Diabet Med.* 2001 Nov;18(11): 871-6.

Veille JC; Sivakoff M; Hanson R; Fanaroff AA. Interventricular septal thickness in fetuses of diabetic mothers. *Obstet Gynecol* 1992;79: 51-4.

Wahabi HA; Alzeidan RA; Bawazeer GA; Alansari LA; Esmaeil SA. Preconception care for diabetic women for improving maternal and fetal outcomes: a systematic review and meta-analysis. *BMC Pregnancy Childbirth*. 2010 Oct 14; 10:63.

Weindling M. Offspring of diabetic pregnancy: short-term outcomes. *Semin Fetal. Neonatal. Med.* 2009 Apr;14(2): 111-8.

Weiss JL; Malone FD; Emig D; Ball RH; Nyberg DA; Comstock CH; Saade G; Eddleman K; Carter SM; Craigo SD; Carr SR; D'Alton ME; FASTER Research Consortium. Obesity, obstetric complications and cesarean delivery rate – a population-based screening study. *Am. J. Obstet. Gynecol.* 2004 Apr;190(4): 1091-7.

Wender-Ozegowska E; Zawiejska A; Ozegowska K; Wroblewska-Seniuk K; Iciek R; Mantai U; Oleiniczak D; Brazert J. Multiple daily injections of insulin versus continuous subcutaneous insulin infusion for pregnant women with type 1 diabetes. *Aust. N. Z. J. Obstet. Gynaecol.* 2013 Apr;53(2): 130-5.

Widness JA; Teramo KA; Clemons GK; Voutilainen P; Stenman UH; McKinlay SM; Schwartz R. Direct relationship of antepartum glucose control and fetal erythropoietin in human type 1 (insulin-dependent) diabetic pregnancy. *Diabetologia.* 1990 Jun;33(6): 378-83.

Wyse LJ; Jones M; Mandel F. Relationship of glycosylated hemoglobin, fetal macrosomia, and birthweight macrosomia. *Am. J. Perinatol.* 1994 Jul;11(4): 260-2.

In: Macrosomia and Birth Weight
Editor: Larry P. Harris

ISBN: 978-1-63483-124-6

Chapter II

Macrosomia and Ambiguous Genitalia: A Review

***Georgios K. Markantes*[1]*, Anastasia K. Armeni*[1]*, Vasiliki Vasileiou*[2] *and Neoklis A. Georgopoulos*[1,*]**

[1]Division of Reproductive Endocrinology,
Department of Obstetrics and Gynecology,
University of Patras Medical School, Patras, Greece
[2]1st Department of Endocrinology, Diabetes Centre,
"Alexandra" Hospital, Athens, Greece

Abstract

Although the concurrence of macrosomia and ambiguous genitalia has been described as early as in the Roman Era (as documented by historian accounts of Titus Livius), such an association remains extremely rare. No obvious correlation between these entities has ever been suggested; still, their non-coincidental contingency sheds light on their intermeshing pathophysiological pathways. Ambiguous genitalia are a surrogate of disorders of sex development (DSD) owing to disorders of gonadal development, inadequate biosynthesis or defective action of sex

* Corresponding and reprint request authors: Neoklis A. Georgopoulos: Department of Obstetrics and Gynecology, Division of Reproductive Endocrinology, University of Patras Medical School, Rio-26500, Greece. Tel:2610-999835, Fax:2610-993854, email: neoklisg@hol.gr.

steroids. Macrosomia is a rather frequent disorder, affecting 1-10% of newborns. Elucidating the variants of birth weight, it has been shown that growth hormone (GH)-related parameters are responsible for up to 40% of the variance of birth weight. Fetal overgrowth syndromes encompassing sexual ambiguity include Beckwith-Wiedemann and Simpson-Golabi-Behmel syndromes, in which distinct phenotypic features are prominently exhibited. Another major growth factor implicated in embryonic development is glucocorticoids. Cortisol overproduction could be a possible causative factor of macrosomia via hyperinsulinemia, which is a major determinant of IGF-I levels. A single defect leading to inappropriate activation of the hypothalamic-pituitary-adrenal (HPA) axis, resulting in cortisol and androgen overproduction could be a possible culprit for the concurrent presence of macrosomia and DSD. Besides, Wilms Tumor 1 (WT1) gene encodes a transcription factor acting as a tumor suppressor protein, while it is implicated in the development of both kidney and early gonad in males. Mutant WT1 protein variants have been shown to inadequately suppress IGF-I receptor promoter activity. Consequently, macrosomia and ambiguous genitalia may be concomitant findings in WT1 related disorders. The aim of the present review is to explore the possible pathophysiological mechanisms whose interplay could result in the co-existence of macrosomia and ambiguous genitalia in neonates.

Keywords: Macrosomia, ambiguous genitalia, pseudohermaphroditism, fetal overgrowth syndromes, Beckwith-Wiedemann syndrome, Simpson-Golabi-Behmel syndrome, Wilms Tumor 1 syndromes, glucocorticoids oveproduction, glucocorticoid resistance, Disorders of Sexual Development (DSD)

Introduction

Although the concurrence of macrosomia and ambiguous genitalia has been described as early as in the Roman Era (as documented by Titus Livius) [1], such an association remains extremely rare. No obvious correlation between these entities has ever been suggested; still, their non-coincidental contingency sheds light on their intermeshing pathophysiological pathways.

After reviewing the pathophysiology of all disorders related to macrosomia and Disorders of Sexual Development (DSD), it was evident that only the rare syndromes Beckwith-Wiedemann and Simpson-Golabi-Behmel, as well as WT1 gene mutations and glucocorticoid receptor defects could possibly lead to an infant with macrosomia and genital ambiguity.

Macrosomia

Human growth ensues from a complex interplay between genetic as well as environmental factors. Macrosomia is associated with numerous maternal as well as neonatal complications and is, therefore, a major cause of adverse pregnancy outcomes [2].

The term macrosomia is used to describe a neonate with excessive birth weight and is diagnosed when the birth weight exceeds a threshold. No universal consensus exists as to which specific threshold should be used when defining macrosomia. Birth weight greater than 4,000 – 4,500g or above the 90th or 97th percentile for gestational age after correcting for neonatal sex and ethnicity are currently in use [3]. The American College of Obstetricians and Gynecologists supports use of the 4500 g threshold for diagnosis of macrosomia because morbidity increases sharply beyond this weight [4].

On the other hand, Liu et al. propose using body mass index (BMI) with a cut-point of 14.2 kg/m^2 in the diagnostic approach, as the evaluation of macrosomia depends not only on the body mass but on the birth length as well [5]. Prevalence apparently depends on diagnostic criteria and it is estimated that macrosomia occurs in 1 – 10% of all deliveries [6]. A constellation of constitutional (multiparity, male sex, advanced maternal age etc) as well as maternal (maternal obesity or diabetes) factors could be responsible for the birth of a macrosomic child [7]. Elevated levels of plasma glucose result in hyperinsulinemia and over expression of insulin-like growth factors (IGFs), which stimulate fetal growth. Besides, McIntyre et al. showed that maternal growth hormone (GH)-related parameters (GH, IGF-I, IGF-II etc) are responsible for up to 40% of the variance of birth weight [8].

A number of rare genetic syndromes are associated with accelerated fetal growth, namely Beckwith-Wiedemann, Simpson-Golabi-Behmel, Pallister-Killian, Sotos, Weaver, Perlman, Costello and Macrocephaly Cutis Marmorata Telangiectasia Congenita. Each one is characterized by distinct phenotypic features; genitourinary malformations have only been described in individuals with Beckwith-Wiedemann and Simpson-Golabi-Behmel syndromes [9, 10].

Ambiguous Genitalia

It is estimated that genital anomalies occur in 1 in 4500 births [11]. Ambiguous genitalia are a phenotypic clue indicating underlying disorders of sex development (DSD). DSD are classified as follows: I) sex chromosome DSD, II) 46,XY DSD and III) 46,XX DSD [11].

Regardless of the karyotype, disorders of gonadal development, excessive or inadequate biosynthesis and/or defective action of sex steroid hormones can explain the vast majority of DSD cases.

The initial stage of gonadal development is identical in both genders. The bipotent gonad emerges at the 4th week of gestation. The differentiation to an ovary or testis begins at the 7th and ends at approximately the 10th week of gestation. Of note, in the bipotent embryonic stage both Wolffian and Müllerian ducts are present; they subsequently regress or differentiate according to the presence or absence of androgens and Anti- Müllerian Hormone (AMH) [12, 13].

This whole process of gonadal development and differentiation is under strict genetic control. Numerous regulatory genes have been identified and clinical syndromes resulting from specific gene mutations have been described [14, 15]. Wilms Tumor suppressor 1 (WT1) and steroidogenic factor 1 (SF-1) genes play a pivotal role in the early stage of indifferent gonad development.

WT1 gene encodes a tumor suppressor protein involved in the development of early gonad and kidney. Mutations lead to gonadal dysgenesis in both sexes (more prominent in 46, XY fetuses) as well as renal anomalies [16-18]. WT1 is also implicated in IGF system activity regulation via interaction with IGF-I receptor promoter and could, therefore, affect fetal growth as well.

SF-1 gene encodes a transcription factor regulating the expression of cytochrome P-450 hydroxylase and 3β-hydroxysteroid dehydrogenase (3β-HSD) enzymes. The phenotypic spectrum of genetic defects in the SF1 gene is broad and depends on the specific mutation [19]. In 46,XY individuals heterozygous mutations in SF-1 may lead to both gonadal and adrenal failure of various degrees [20, 21], while ovarian development seems to be affected in a much lesser degree [22].

The importance of a number of other genes (EMX2, M33, LHX9 and GATA4) in the development of the bipotent gonad has been proven in mice, but not yet in humans [23].

Four genes are indispensable for ovarian differentiation. WNT4 gene is essential for nephrogenesis, inhibition of enzymes responsible for androgen synthesis and formation of Müllerian duct structures [24]. DAX1 gene mediates SRY inactivation in females, while promoting spermatogenesis in males [25, 26]. FOXL2 gene has a crucial role in ovarian development and maintenance; mutations lead to female-to-male sex reversal in animals, while in humans cause premature ovarian failure [27, 28]. The RSPO1 gene appears to be directly involved in ovarian determination as mutations have been associated with 46,XX testicular and ovotesticular DSD [29].

Sex-determining region on the Y chromosome (SRY) and SOX9 genes are the major determinants of testicular development, allowing testis cords and Sertoli cells differentiation [30]. Malfunction of these genes leads to 46,XY DSD, whereas inappropriate expression in 46,XX individuals has been shown to cause 46,XX testicular and ovotesticular DSD [31-33].

Desert hedgehog protein (DHH) and PDGFRA genes are important in Leydig cell differentiation; mutations cause testicular dysgenesia [34]. Finally, mutations in ATRX and ARX genes may also lead to dysgenetic testes [11].

Various enzymatic defects in the cascade of steroidogenesis can result in either excessive or inadequate synthesis of sex steroids. Numerous mutations of genes encoding key enzymes have been identified. Examples include: StAR (congenital lipoid adrenal hyperplasia), CYP11B1, CYP21A2 & HSD3B2 (congenital adrenal hyperplasia – CAH), P450 Oxidoreductase, CYP17 and SRD5A2 (5a reductase deficiency) [11].

Finally, mutations altering the responsiveness of steroid hormones receptors lead to conditions of sex steroid insensitivity, rendering target-tissues irresponsive to hormonal action. Defects in Androgen, AMH and glucocorticoid receptors causing DSD have been described [11].

After reviewing the pathophysiology of all the aforementioned disorders, it was evident that only WT1 gene mutations and glucocorticoid receptor defects could possibly lead to macrosomia besides DSD.

Beckwith-Wiedemann Syndrome

Beckwith-Wiedemann syndrome (BWS) was first described in the 1960's, when Hans-Rudolf Wiedemann in Germany and J.B. Beckwith in the USA reported a series of patients presenting with congenital exomphalos, macroglossia and gigantism. BWS is the most common overgrowth syndrome in infancy and also carries a predisposition to tumor development [35]. It is characterized by phenotypic variability as well as etiologic molecular heterogeneity.

Prevalence is estimated to be 1:13, 700 live births [36]. It usually occurs sporadically (85%), whereas in 15% of cases familial transmission –most commonly autosomal dominant with variable expressivity- has been observed. The incidence is equal in males and females; several reports indicate increased frequency in IVF infants, while others do not support this finding. In a recent review using data from 8 epidemiological studies, the authors calculated a RR of 5.2 (95% CI 1.6-7.4) for BWS after IVF/ICSI compared with naturally conceived children, and of 4.0 (95% CI 2.0-8.3) for assisted reproduction techniques (ART) other than IVF/ICSI. Whether ART are themselves the cause of the increased incidence of BWS or other factors (e.g., parental genetic background) are responsible remains to be proven [37].

The BWS region of the short arm of chromosome 11 was the first identified example of genomic imprinting in humans. This process refers to the monoallelic expression of a gene in a parent-of-origin specific manner. Genomic imprinting is regulated by epigenetic mechanisms (extrinsic to changes in primary nucleotide sequence) that include DNA methylation, histone modification, and noncoding RNAs [38]. In healthy individuals, only the maternal or paternal allele of a number of genes on 11p15.5 is expressed (imprinted allele). Abnormal regulation of gene expression in this chromosomal region can lead to biallelic expression and dysregulation of pre- and postnatal growth [39-41].

There are four critical growth regulatory genes associated with genomic imprinting in chromosome 11p15: Insulin-like growth factor II (IGF-II) - a major growth factor in utero [42], H19 - a tumor suppressor and growth restrictor [43, 44], CDKN1C - a cyclin-dependent kinase inhibitor that down-regulates cell proliferation [45] and KCNQ10T1 – a CDKN1C inhibitor [46].

A number of different molecular mechanisms can lead to BWS via either epigenetic or genetic alterations in the chromosome 11p15.5 genes mentioned above. These modifications change the relative contributions of parental alleles resulting in over expression of growth promoting and/or under expression of growth suppressing genes [39-41]. A molecular alteration in 11p15.5 is identified in only 75-80% of patients with BWS [38]. This may be due, in part, to somatic mosaicism for some of the molecular alterations but other genomic loci are probably involved in the pathogenesis of BWS [47-49].

The hallmark features of BWS are omphalocele, macroglossia and macrosomia; however, it is characterized by significant phenotypic heterogeneity [50] and correlations between clinical findings and specific molecular defects exist [38]. A recognizable facial gestalt is common [36] and visceromegaly involving one or more intra-abdominal organs may be present. Neonatal hypoglycemia is reported in up to 50% of cases and it is likely secondary to islet cell hyperplasia and hyperinsulinemia [36, 51]. Mental retardation has been reported and is most likely secondary to uncontrolled hypoglycemia during infancy. Cytomegaly of the fetal adrenal cortex is pathognomonic when present [9], while renal manifestations (primary malformations, nephrocalcinosis etc) are commonly described [52-54]. Other features include cleft palate, cardiomegaly, cardiomyopathy, diastasis recti, advanced bone age and genital malformations [9].

Of major concern in children with BWS is the predisposition to embryonal tumors: Wilm's tumor and hepatoblastoma are the most common and the overall tumor risk is estimated to be between 4 and 21% [55-57].

Many cases of patients with BWS presenting with signs of virilization developing in childhood, adolescence or even early adulthood are described in the literature. Androgen-producing adrenocortical tumors are the cause of such presentations [58-61]. Clitoromegaly may be present (along with acne, voice change, excessive hair growth), especially in tumors affecting young girls [59]. However, an adrenal tumor cannot account for genital ambiguity in a newborn. The concurrence of BWS with 46,XX ovotesticular DSD was only recently reported for the first time [62]. It was a Mexican girl with typical features of BWS, clitoromegaly, undersized vaginal introitus and hypoplastic labia. Cytogenic analysis revealed a 46,XX karyotype and no Y chromosome sequences were identified with FISH. Gonadal histology studies proved the presence of ovotestes. The authors propose two possible mechanisms to explain the co-existence of BWS and DSD: a concurrent mutation in WT1 gene which is located in 11p13 -relatively close to the BWS region in 11p15- or a modification in ZAC1 transcription factor which regulates the expression of genes implicated both in BWS (IGF-II and H19) and in gonadal development (SOX11) [63, 64]. The IGF system seems indeed to be the most promising area for research for a common pathophysiological path connecting BWS and ambiguous genitalia. IGF-I, IGF-II, IGF binding proteins 1 and 3, GH and GH binding protein are strongly correlated with birth weight [8], while the differentiation, mitogenesis and steroidogenesis of rat Leydig cells - the testosterone producing cells- are enhanced by IGF-I & IGF-II signaling pathways [65].

Simpson-Golabi-Behmel Syndrome

Simpson-Golabi-Behmel syndrome (SGBS) is an overgrowth / multiple congenital anomalies X-linked disorder. It was first reported during the 1970's and named by Neri et al. in the late 1980's [66]. Pre- and postnatal overgrowth, characteristic facies and abnormalities of the skeleton and internal organs are the most consistent features, as is the association with embryonal tumors [10].

The exact prevalence of SGBS is unknown. It is a rare disorder; to date, about 250 patients have been reported in the literature [10].

There are two distinct subtypes of the syndrome: the classical SGBS or SGBS type I and a very infrequent lethal form or SGBS type II (with less than 10 cases described, all dying within the first weeks of life) [67, 68].

SGBS is an X-linked disorder and, as such, males baring the mutant gene in their only X chromosome express the phenotype while females are only carriers of the disease. Some female carriers may exhibit mild physical findings of SGBS (Lyonization phenomenon).

SGBS type I is caused by mutations involving the glypican-3 (GPC3) gene, located in Xq26.2. Glypican-3 is a cell surface heparin sulfate proteoglycan which regulates signaling pathways implicated in cell division and growth regulation. Point mutations, dislocations and duplications resulting in loss of function of GPC3 have been reported in SGBS patients.

SGBS is characterized by macrosomia and macrocephaly associated with craniosynostosis in the majority of cases. Facial traits are "coarse" and typically include cleft lip and/or palate, macrostomia, macroglossia, hypertelorism, dental malocclusion, epicanthal folds and downslanting palpebral fissures. Supernumerary nipples are frequently present, not only in males but in female carriers as well. Multiple congenital anomalies are usually present and may involve the cardiovascular system, gastrointestinal tract, central nervous system, skeleton and genitalia (hypospadias, chryptorchidism). Visceromegaly is also common and affects the kidneys, liver and spleen, while diaphragmatic hernia has also been reported [10, 69].

Affected individuals are considered to be at increased risk for tumor development. Wilm's tumor and hepatoblastoma are the commonest and usually appear within the first decade of life, while other tumors have also been described [57]. In SGBS, genitalia are usually normal although hypospadias, cryptorchidism and penoscrotal transposition have been reported [70]. A recent case report describes a patient with a frameshift mutation in

GPC3 presenting with penoscrotal hypospadias and a large prostatic urticle (recorded for the first time in SGBS); low levels of cortisol and testosterone were also noticed [71], suggesting adrenal and gonadal dysfunction. A possible link between overgrowth and genital ambiguity in SGBS can be sought in the pattern of expression of GPC3 as well as in its regulating action over important genes involved in gonadal development. GPC3 expression is highly tissue- and stage-specific during gestation. In the genital system, GPC3 is homogenously but weekly expressed in early pregnancy prior to gonadal differentiation. In contrast, later in gestation, the testis, epidydimis, vas deferens and male urethra are strongly positive for GPC3 expression, while female structures are negative [72]. Hence, glypican-3 seems to be an indispensable component for normal development and function of the testis.

Given the critical role of IGF-II in human growth and the proven association of IGF-II dysregulation with overgrowth syndromes (such as Beckwith-Wiedemann syndrome), it was initially thought that glypican-3 was an inhibitor of IGF-II and that the overgrowth observed in SGBS was due to an increase in IGF-II signaling. However, studies in rats have shown that GPC3 does not interact with IGF-II and that GPC3-null embryos display normal levels of IGF-II [73, 74]. Furthermore, experiments in double mutant mice lacking GPC3 and also IGF-II, IGF-I, or the type 1 IGF receptor (IGF1R) provided conclusive genetic evidence inconsistent with the hypothesis that GPC3 acts as a growth suppressor by sequestering or downregulating an IGF ligand [75]. Instead, studies in mice as well as in Drosophila cells have demonstrated that glypican-3 inhibits the hedgehog signaling pathway, a very important promoter of embryonic cell growth and proper development acting in many tissues [76, 77]. Hyperactivation of hedgehog signaling caused by the loss of functional glypican-3 explains the overgrowth and congenital anomalies found in SGBS. Of note, desert hedgehog protein (DHH) -one of the three proteins of the hedgehog family found in mammals- has a cardinal role in Leydig cell differentiation. Mutations of DHH can even lead to testicular dysgenesia [34]. It is therefore possible that a dysregulation of DHH signaling due to a mutant GPC3 gene might be responsible for the genital anomalies seen in SGBS.

Wilms Tumor 1 (WT1) Gene Mutations

WT1 gene is located at chromosome 11p13 and encodes a zinc finger motif-containing protein acting as a transcription factor. Apart from its role in initiating or promoting Wilms tumor, it is also involved in genitourinary development [78].

A multitude of different isoforms (up to 24) of WT1 protein may result from a combination of alternative translational start sites, alternative RNA splicing, and RNA editing [79]. Different isoforms seem to have overlapping but also distinct functions. For example, alternative splicing affecting exon 9 allows the insertion or exclusion of three amino acids [lysine-threonine-serine (KTS)] between zinc fingers 3 and 4. Variants lacking KTS (-KTS) bind to DNA and act as transcriptional regulators, while KTS containing isoforms (+KTS) have higher affinity for RNA and act at the post-transcriptional level. The ratio of splice variants is highly conserved and alterations have been linked to specific diseases [80].

Certain loss-of-function mutations of WT1 gene result in a spectrum of disorders, namely Frasier, Denys-Drash and WAGR syndromes. These syndromes are characterized by renal disease, genital ambiguity and predisposition to tumorigenesis [81]. With respect to genital abnormalities, sexes are unequally affected: 46,XY fetuses present as male pseudohermaphrodites with ambiguous or female external genitalia due to testicular dysgenesia, while in 46,XX individuals the phenotype is usually normal as gonads are only occasionally affected [18]. Renal manifestations include diffuse mesangial sclerosis and nephrotic syndrome rapidly progressing in end-stage renal disease in Denys-Drash syndrome; slowly progressing nephrotic syndrome and focal segmental glomerulosclerosis in Frasier syndrome. Individuals with Denys-Drash syndrome are at increased risk for Wilms tumor, whereas a high incidence of gonadoblastoma is observed in patients with Frasier syndrome [79]. Finally, WAGR syndrome is characterized by Wilms tumor, Aniridia, Genitourinary malformations and mental Retardation [81]. Of note, macrosomia is not included in the phenotypic “mosaic” of any of the aforementioned syndromes.

As mentioned before, maternal GH-related parameters are responsible for up to 40% of the variance of birth weight [8]. It has been shown that in the 2nd half of gestation maternal pituitary GH is progressively replaced by placental GH, which is a major determinant of maternal IGF-I levels [82, 83]. As GH is unable to cross the placenta, its somatogenic effects on the fetus are most likely mediated by IGFs.

IGF-I and IGF-II exert the majority of their biological actions via IGF-I receptor (IGF-I-R). In vitro studies by Werner et al. have demonstrated a solid correlation between WT1 and IGF-I-R, showing that a major aspect of WT1 protein action is the suppression of IGF-I-R promoter activity (via binding to multiple binding sites) and, thus, suppression of IGF-I-R expression [84, 85].

Moreover, WT1 gene product is able to bind to RNA of the insulin-like growth factor-2 gene, as part of its post-transcriptional actions [79].

Consequently, mutations in WT1 could theoretically cause macrosomia besides ambiguous genitalia via increased IGF-I and/or IGF-II activity. A possible reason why macrosomia is not a consistent finding in carriers of such mutations might be sought in the wide variety of isoforms of WT1 protein: different variants likely suppress IGF activity to a different extent with macrosomia being a consequence only in mutations leading to loss of function of highly suppressive variants.

Cortisol Production Disorders

Glucocorticoids regulate a broad spectrum of physiologic functions essential for life. Besides their fundamental role in maintaining homeostasis, they have been shown to be among the principal variants of fetal development (CNS, lungs etc) and growth [86]. Increased circulating glucose levels is the cardinal metabolic effect of glucocorticoid activity either via increased glucose production (stimulation of hepatic gluconeogenesis or increased breakdown of muscle and fat to provide additional substrates for glucose production) or through inhibition of insulin release from pancreatic β cells leading to decreased peripheral glucose uptake. However, hyperglycaemia is compensated by increased insulin secretion, resulting in hyperinsulinemia and insulin resistance [87]. Given the link between increased insulin and high IGF-I levels, as well as the correlation of IGF-I with fetal macrosomia, disorders leading to cortisol overproduction could be a causative factor of macrosomia via hyperinsulinemia.

Increased androgen levels in utero cause virilization of female fetuses. Various cortisol production disorders resulting in androgen excess lead to 46,XX newborns exhibiting ambiguous genitalia characterized by clitoral enlargement, fusion of the labial folds and rostral migration of the urethral/vaginal perineal orifice [88]. Despite the fact that androgens accelerate growth and bone maturation in childhood, their impact on birth weight appears to be minimal [89].

Any condition leading to inappropriate activation of the hypothalamic-pituitary-adrenal (HPA) axis during fetal life and, hence, overproduction of glucocorticoids and androgens, could be a possible culprit for the concurrent presence of macrosomia and genital ambiguity in 46,XX neonates. In fact, in generalised glucocorticoid resistance, certain mutations in the glucocorticoid receptor gene prevent glucocorticoids from exerting their actions on target tissues. Abolishment of cortisol-mediated negative feedback leads to activation of the HPA axis. The excess ACTH secretion results in adrenal hyperplasia and increased production of cortisol along with increased mineralocorticoid activity (due to overproduction of cortisol, deoxycorticosterone and corticosterone), as well as androgen excess (due to overproduction of androstenedione, dehydroepiandrosterone, and dehydroepiandrosterone-sulfate (DHEAS)). The phenotype comprises ambiguous genitalia at birth in females and later on signs of androgen and mineralocorticoid excess in both sexes [90, 91].

Notwithstanding, aberrant fetal growth has never been reported in generalised glucocorticoid resistance – a rather expected finding as glucocorticoids are unable to significantly increase glucose due to target tissue (liver, muscle, adipose) insensitivity. However, a theoretical defect causing glucocorticoid resistance confined only in some tissues (e.g., hypothalamus) while sparing others could lead to macrosomia besides DSD.

Finally, when examining cortisol production disorders, one should also consider the fetal adrenal cortex physiology. As part of the fetoplacental unit, fetal adrenal cortex is the major contributor to estradiol production after the 8th week of gestation. Estradiol, which is essential for maintenance of pregnancy, is produced in the placenta, using DHEAS from the fetal adrenals as the main substrate. Hence, DHEAS is secreted by fetal adrenals in large amounts being the main adrenal steroid in gestation [92]. However, during the critical period of sexual differentiation (7th – 10th week of gestation) cortisol biosynthesis by the fetal adrenal cortex temporarily suppresses the HPA axis and prevents excessive androgen production, protecting female fetuses from virilization [93]. Cortisol secretion then decreases, to be increased again only in late gestation, when it is essential for lung maturation and parturition [92].

Furthermore, 3βHSD, the enzyme converting pregnenolone to progesterone, is avidly expressed only in late pregnancy while data regarding its earlier expression is conflicting [93], suggesting that it represents the key site of control with respect to fetal cortisol biosynthesis during pregnancy. Consequently, the timing of cortisol action in utero makes a prominent effect on fetal growth rather unlikely and macrosomia of glucocorticoid overproduction origin a remote possibility.

References

[1] Vasileiou, V; Armeni, AK; Pierris, AL; Georgopoulos, NA. Macrosomia and ambiguous genitalia: a long overdue answer to the citizens of Frusino.. *Hormones* (Athens) 2012;11(2): 215-221.

[2] Ju, H; Chadha, Y; Donovan, T; O'Rourke, P. Fetal macrosomia and pregnancy outcomes. *Aust N Z J Obstet Gynaecol* 2009;49(5): 504-509.

[3] Ye, J; Zhang, L; Chen, Y; Fang, F; Luo, Z; et al. Searching for the Definition of Macrosomia through an Outcome-Based Approach. *PLOS ONE,* 2014;9(6): e100192. doi:10.1371.

[4] ACOG Practice Bulletin No 22: Fetal Macrosomia. American College of Obstetricians and Gynecologists, Washington DC, 2000.

[5] Liu, XX; Song, WW; Liu, HB. Evaluation the significance of body mass index in diagnosing macrosomia in human neonate. *Zhonghua Fu Chan Ke Za Zhi* 2010;45(7): 488-491.

[6] Martin, JA; Hamilton, BE; Sutton, PD; Ventura, SJ; Menacker, F; Kirmeyer, S. Births: final data for 2004. *Natl Vital Stat Rep* 2006;55(1): 1-101.

[7] Okun, N; Verma, A; Mitchell, BF; Flowerdew, G. Relative importance of maternal constitutional factors and glucose intolerance of pregnancy in the development of newborn macrosomia. *J Matern Fetal Med* 1997;6(5): 285-290.

[8] Mcintyre, HD; Serek, R; Crane, DI; et al. Placental Growth Hormone (GH), GH-Binding Protein, and insulin-like Growth Factor Axis in Normal, Growth-retarded, and Diabetic Pregnancies: Correlations with Fetal Growth. *J Clin Endocrinol Metab* 2000;85(3): 1143-1150.

[9] Shuman, C; Smith, AC; Weksberg, R. Beckwith-Wiedemann syndrome. *Gene Reviews* [Internet] 2008.

[10] Tenorio, J; Arias, P; Martínez-Glez, V; Santos, F; García-Miñaur, S; Nevado, J; Lapunzina, P. Simpson-golabi-behmel syndrome types I and II. Orphanet *J Rare Dis* 2014;9(1): 138 [Epub ahead of print].

[11] Hughes, IA; Houk, C; Ahmed, SF; Lee, PA; LWPES1/ESPE2 Consensus Group. Consensus statement on management of intersex disorders. *Arch Dis Child* 2006;91: 554–562.

[12] Sadler, TW. Third to eight weeks: The embryonic period. In: Lippincott Williams & Wilkins, editors. *Langman's Medical Embryology* 10th edition. Baltimore, Maryland, USA; 2006; pp 67-87.

[13] Sadler, TW. Urogenital system. In: Lippincott Williams & Wilkins, editors. *Langman's Medical Embryology* 10th edition. Baltimore, Maryland, USA; 2006; pp 229-256.

[14] Maclaughlin, DT; Donahoe, PK. Sex determination and differentiation. N Engl J Med 2004;350: 367-378.

[15] Hughes, IA. Female Development – All by Default? *N Engl J Med* 2004;351: 748-750.

[16] Jaubert, F; Vasiliu, V; Patey-Mariaud de Serre, N; et al. Gonad development in Drash and Frasier syndromes depends on WT1 mutations. *Arkh Patol* 2003;65: 40-44.

[17] Demmer, L; Primack, W; Loik, V; Brown, R; Therville, N; McElreavey, K. Frasier syndrome: a cause of focal segmental glomerulosclerosis in a 46,XX female. *J Am Soc Nephrol* 1999;10: 2215-2218.

[18] Koziell, A; Grundy, R. Frasier and Denys-Drash syndromes: different disorders or part of a spectrum? *Arch Dis Child* 1999;81: 365-369.

[19] Lin, L; Achermann, JC. Steroidogenic factor-1 (SF-1, Ad4BP, NR5A1) and disorders of testis development. *Sex Dev* 2008;2: 200-209.

[20] Mallet, D; Bretones, P; Michel-Calemard, L; Dijoud, F; David, M; Morel, Y. Gonadal dysgenesis without adrenal insufficiency in a46,XY patient heterozygous for the nonsense C16X mutation: a case of SF1 haploinsufficiency. *J Clin Endocrinol Metab* 2004;89: 4829-4832.

[21] Achermann, JC; Ito, M; Ito, M; Hindmarsh, PC; Jameson, JL. A mutation in the gene encoding steroidogenic factor-1 causes XY sex reversal and adrenal failure in humans. *Nat Genet* 1999;22: 125-126.

[22] Biason-Lauber, A; Schoenle, EJ. Apparently normal ovarian differentiation in a prepubertal girl with transcriptionally inactive steroidogenic factor 1 (NR5A1/SF-1) and adrenocortical insufficiency. *Am J Hum Genet* 2000;67(6): 1563-1568.

[23] Wilhelm, D; Palmer, S; Koopman, P. Sex determination and gonadal development in mammals. *Physiol Rev* 2007;87: 1-28.

[24] Morcel, K; Camborieux, L; Programme de recherches sur les Aplasies Müllériennes; Guerrier, D. Mayer-Rokitansky-Küster-Hauser (MRKH) syndrome. *Orphanet J Rare Dis* 2007;2: 13.

[25] Yu, RN; Ito, M; Saunders, TL; Camper, SA; Jameson, JL. Role of Ahch in gonadal development and gametogenesis. *Nat Genet* 1998;20: 353-357.

[26] Mizusaki, H; Kawabe, K; Mukai, T; et al. Dax-1 (dosage-sensitive sex reversal-adrenal hypoplasia congenital critical region on the X chromosome, gene 1) gene transcription is regulated by wnt4 in the female developing gonad. *Mol Endocrinol* 2003;17: 507-519.

[27] Pailhoux, E; Vigier, B; Vaiman, D; et al. Ontogenesis of female-to-male sex-reversal in XX polled goats. *Dev Dyn* 2002;224(1): 39-50.

[28] Beysen, D; Vandesompele, J; Messiaen, L; De Paepe, A; De Baere, E. The human FOXL2 mutation database. *Hum Mutat* 2004;24: 189-193.

[29] Tomaselli, S; Megiorni, F; De Bernardo, C; et al. Syndromic true hermaphroditism due to an R-spondin1 (RSPO1) homozygous mutation. *Hum Mutat* 2008;29: 220-226.

[30] Brennan, J; Capel, B. One tissue, two fates: molecular genetic events that underlie testis versus ovary development. *Nat Rev Genet* 2004;5(7): 509-521.

[31] Ortenberg, J; Oddoux, C; Craver, R; et al. SRY gene expression in the ovotestes of XX true hermaphrodites. *J Urol* 2002;167: 1828-1831.

[32] López, M; Torres, L; Méndez, JP; et al. Clinical traits and molecular findings in 46, XX males. *Clin Genet* 1995;48: 29-34.

[33] Huang, B; Wang, S; Ning, Y; Lamb, AN; Bartley, J. Autosomal XX sex reversal caused by duplication of SOX9. *Am J Med Genet* 1999;87: 349-353.

[34] Griswold, SL; Behringer, RR. Fetal Leydig cell origin and development. *Sex Dev* 2009;3: 1-15.

[35] Spivey, PS; Bradshaw, WT. Recognition and management of the infant with Beckwith-Wiedemann Syndrome. *Adv Neonatal Care* 2009;9(6): 279-284.

[36] Pettenati, MJ; Haines, JL; Higgins, RR; Wappner, RS; Palmer, CG; Weaver, DD. Wiedemann-Beckwith syndrome: presentation of clinical and cytogenetic data on 22 new cases and review of the literature. *Hum Genet* 1986;74(2): 143-154.

[37] Vermeiden, JP; Bernardus RE. Are imprinting disorders more prevalent after human in vitro fertilization or intracytoplasmic sperm injection? *Fertil Steril* 2013;99(3): 642-651.

[38] Weksberg, R; Shuman, C; Beckwith, JB. Beckwith-Wiedemann syndrome. *Eur J Hum Genet* 2010;18(1): 8-14.

[39] Cooper, WN; Luharia, A; Evans, GA; et al. Molecular subtypes and phenotypic expression of Beckwith-Wiedemann syndrome. *Eur J Hum Genet* 2005;13(9): 1025-1032.

[40] Enklaar, T; Zabel, BU; Prawitt, D. Beckwith-Wiedemann syndrome: multiple molecular mechanisms. *Expert Rev Mol Med* 2006;8(17): 1-19.

[41] Weksberg, R; Shuman, C; Smith, AC. Beckwith-Wiedemann syndrome. *Am J Med Genet C Semin Med Genet* 2005;137C(1): 12-23.

[42] Ko, JM. Genetic syndromes associated with overgrowth in childhood. *Ann Pediatr Endocrinol Metab* 2013;18(3): 101-105.

[43] Hao, Y; Crenshaw, T; Moulton, T; Newcomb, E; Tycko, B. Tumour-suppressor activity of H19 RNA. *Nature* 1993;365: 764-767.

[44] Guo, L; Choufani, S; Ferreira, J; Smith, A; Chitayat, D; Shuman, C; et al. Altered gene expression and methylation of the human chromosome 11 imprinted region in small for gestational age (SGA) placentae. *Dev Biol* 2008;320: 79-91.

[45] Tsugu, A; Sakai, K; Dirks, PB; Jung, S; Weksberg, R; Fei, YL; et al. Expression of p57(KIP2) potently blocks the growth of human astrocytomas and induces cell senescence. *Am J Pathol* 2000;157: 919-932.

[46] Cerrato, F; Vernucci, M; Pedone, PV; Chiariotti, L; Sebastio, G; Bruni, CB; et al. The 5' end of the KCNQ1OT1 gene is hypomethylated in the Beckwith-Wiedemann syndrome. *Hum Genet* 2002;111: 105-107.

[47] Meyer, E; Lim, D; Pasha, S; et al. Germline mutation in NLRP2 (NALP2) in a familial imprinting disorder (Beckwith-Wiedemann Syndrome). *PLoS Genet* 2009;5(3): e1000423. doi: 10.1371.

[48] Mackay, DJ; Callaway, JL; Marks, SMet al. Hypomethylation of multiple imprinted loci in individuals with transient neonatal diabetes is associated with mutations in ZFP57. *Nat Genet* 2008;40(8): 949-951.

[49] Naik, S; Riordan-Eva, E; Thomas, NS; Poole, R; Ashton, M; Crolla, JA; Temple, IK. Large de novo deletion of 7p15.1 to 7p12.1 involving the imprinted gene GRB10 associated with a complex phenotype including features of Beckwith Wiedemann syndrome. *Eur J Med Genet* 2011;54(1): 89-93.

[50] Beckwith, JB. Extreme cytomegaly of the adrenal fetal cortex, omphalocele, hyperplasia of kidneys and pancreas, and Leydig-cell hyperplasia: Another syndrome? *Western Society for Pediatric Research* (Ed), Los Angeles; 1963.

[51] Engstrom, W; Lindham, S; Schofield, P. Wiedemann–Beckwith syndrome. *Eur J Pediatri* 1988;147: 450–457.

[52] Choyke, PL; Siegel, MJ; Oz, O; Sotelo-Avila, C; De Baum, MR. Nonmalignant renal disease in pediatric patients with Beckwith–Wiedemann syndrome. *AJR Am J Roentgenol* 1998;171: 733–737.

[53] Borer, JG; Kaefer, M; Barnwolt, CE; et al. Renal findings on radiological follow-up of patients with Beckwith–Wiedemann syndrome. *J Urol* 1999;161: 235–239.

[54] Goldman, M; Smith, A; Shuman, C; et al. Renal abnormalities in Beckwith–Wiedemann syndrome are associated with 11p15.5 uniparental disomy. *J Am Soc Nephrol* 2002;13: 2077–2084.

[55] Tan, TY; Amor, DJ. Tumour surveillance in Beckwith–Wiedemann syndrome and hemihyperplasia: a critical review of the evidence and suggested guidelines for local practice. *J Paed Child Health* 2006;42: 486–490.

[56] Sotelo-Avila, C; Gonzalex-Crussi, F; Fowler, JW. Complete and incomplete forms of Beckwith–Wiedemann syndrome: their oncogenic potential. *J Pediatr* 1980;96: 47–50.

[57] Lapunzina, P. Risk of tumorigenesis in overgrowth syndromes: a comprehensive review. *Am J Med Genet* 2005;137: 53–71.

[58] Bertoin, F; Letouzé, E; Grignani, P; et al. Genome-Wide Paternal Uniparental Disomy as a Cause of Beckwith-Wiedemann Syndrome Associated with Recurrent Virilizing Adrenocortical Tumors. *Horm Metab Res* 2014 Nov 3 [Epub ahead of print].

[59] Mizota, M; Tamada, I; Hizukuri, K; et al. Bilateral asynchronous adrenocortical adenoma in a girl with beckwith-wiedemann syndrome. *Clin Pediatr Endocrinol* 2005;14(1): 23-26.

[60] Sbragia-Neto, L; Melo-Filho, AA; Guerra-Júnior, G; et al. Beckwith-Wiedemann syndrome and virilizing cortical adrenal tumor in a child. *J Pediatr Surg* 2000;35(8): 1269-1271.

[61] Clouston, WM; Cannell, GC; Fryar, BG; Searle, JW; Martin, NI; Mortimer, RH. Virilizing adrenal adenoma in an adult with the Beckwith-Wiedemann syndrome: paradoxical response to dexamethasone. *Clin Endocrinol* (Oxf) 1989;31(4): 467-473.

[62] Macías-Gómez, NM; Leal-Ugarte, E; Gutiérrez-Angulo, M; Domínguez-Quezada, G; Rivera, H; Barros-Núñez, P. 46,XX ovotesticular disorder in a Mexican patient with Beckwith-Wiedemann syndrome: a case report. *J Med Case Rep* 2012;6: 301.

[63] Tsuda, T; Markova, D; Wang, H; Evangelisti, L; Pan, TC; Chu, ML. Zinc finger protein Zac1 is expressed in chondrogenic sites of the mouse. *Dev Dyn* 2004;229(2): 340-348.

[64] Zhang, L; Lin, D; Zhang, Y; Ma, G; Zhang, W. A homologue of Sox11 predominantly expressed in the ovary of the orange-spotted grouper Epinephelus coioides. *Comp Biochem Physiol B Biochem Mol Biol* 2008;149(2): 345-353.

[65] Colón, E; Zaman, F; Axelson, M; et al. Insulin-Like Growth Factor-I is an Important Antiapoptotic Factor for Rat Leydig Cells during Postnatal Development. *Endocrinology* 2007;148: 128-139.

[66] Neri, G; Marini, R; Cappa, M; Borrelli, P; Opitz, JM. Simpson-Golabi-Behmel syndrome: an X-linked encephalo-tropho-schisis syndrome. *Am J Med Genet* 1988;30: 287–299.

[67] Brzustowicz, LM; Farrell, S; Khan, MB; Weksberg, R. Mapping of a new SGBS locus to chromosome Xp22 in a family with a severe form of Simpson-Golabi-Behmel syndrome. *Am J Hum Genet* 1999;65: 779–783.

[68] Terespolsky, D; Farrell, SA; Siegel-Bartelt, J; Weksberg, R. Infantile lethal variant of Simpson-Golabi-Behmel syndrome associated with hydrops fetalis. *Am J Med Genet* 1995;59: 329–333.

[69] Neri, G; Gurrieri, F; Zanni, G; Lin, A. Clinical and molecular aspects of the Simpson-Golabi-Behmel syndrome. *Am J Med Genet.* 1998;79(4): 279-283.

[70] Griffith, CB; Probert, RC; Vance, GH. Genital anomalies in three male siblings with Simpson-Golabi-Behmel syndrome. *Am J Med Genet A* 2009;149A: 2484–2488.

[71] Villarreal, DD; Villarreal, H; Paez, AM; Peppas, D; Lynch, J; Roeder, E; Powers, GC. A patient with a unique frameshift mutation in GPC3, causing Simpson-Golabi-Behmel syndrome, presenting with craniosynostosis, penoscrotal hypospadias, and a large prostatic utricle. *Am J Med Genet* 2013;161A(12): 3121-3125.

[72] Iglesias, BV; Centeno, G; Pascuccelli, H; et al. Expression pattern of glypican-3 (GPC3) during human embryonic and fetal development. Histol Histopathol 2008;23: 1333-1340.

[73] Cano-Gauci, DF; Song, HH; Yang, H; et al. Glypican-3-deficient mice exhibit developmental overgrowth and some of the abnormalities typical of Simpson-Golabi-Behmel syndrome. *J Cell Biol* 1999;146: 255–264.

[74] Song, HH; Shi, W; Filmus, J. OCI-5/rat glypican-3 binds to fibroblast growth factor-2 but not to insulin-like growth factor-2. *J Biol Chem* 1997;272: 7574–7577.

[75] Chiao, E; Fisher, P; Crisponi, L; Deiana, M; Dragatsis, I; Schlessinger, D; Pilia, G; Efstratiadis, A. Overgrowth of a mouse model of the

Simpson-Golabi-Behmel syndrome is independent of IGF signaling. *Dev Biol* 2002;243: 185–206.

[76] Capurro, MI; Xu, P; Shi, W; Li, F; Jia, A; Filmus, J. Glypican-3 inhibits Hedgehog signaling during development by competing with patched for Hedgehog binding. *Dev Cell* 2008;14: 700–711.

[77] Williams, EH; Pappano, WN; Saunders, AM; Kim, MS; Leahy, DJ; Beachy, PA. Dally-like core protein and its mammalian homologues mediate stimulatory and inhibitory effects on Hedgehog signal response. *Proc Natl Acad Sci USA* 2010;107: 5869–5874.

[78] Pritchard-Jones, K; Fleming, S; Davidson, D; et al. The candidate Wilms' tumour gene is involved in genitourinary development. *Nature* 1990;346: 194-197.

[79] Mrowka, C; Schedl, A. Wilms' tumor suppressor gene WT1: from structure to renal pathophysiologic features. *J Am Soc Nephrol* 2000;11 Suppl 16:S106-115.

[80] Laity, JH; Chung, J; Dyson, HJ; Wright, PE. Alternative splicing of Wilms' tumour suppressor protein modulates DNA binding activity through isoform-specific DNA-induced conformational changes. *Biochemistry* 2000;39: 5341-5348.

[81] Andrade, JG; Guaragna, MS; Soardi, FC; Guerra-Júnior, G; Mello, MP; Maciel-Guerra, AT. Clinical and genetic findings of five patients with WT1-related disorders. *Arq Bras Endocrinol Metabol* 2008;52(8): 1236-1243.

[82] Frankenne, F; Closset, J; Gomez, F; Scippo, ML; Smal, J; Hennen, G. The physiology of growth hormones (GHs) in pregnant women and partial characterization of the placental GH variant. *J Clin Endocrinol Metab* 1988;66: 1171-1180.

[83] Caufriez, A; Frankenne, F; Englert, Y; et al. Placental growth hormone as a potential regulator of maternal IGF-I during human pregnancy. *Am J Physiol* 1990;258: E1014-E1019.

[84] Werner, H; Rauscher III, FJ; Sukhatme, VP; Drummond, IA; Roberts Jr, CT; LeRoith, D. Transcriptional repression of the insulin-like growth factor I receptor (IGF-I-R) gene by the tumor suppressor WT1 involves binding to sequences both upstream and downstream of the IGF-I-R gene transcription start site. *J Biol Chem* 1994;269: 12577-12582.

[85] Werner, H; Shen-Orr, Z; Rauscher III, FJ; Morris, JF; Roberts Jr, CT; LeRoith, D. Inhibition of cellular proliferation by the Wilms' tumor suppressor WT1 is associated with suppression of insulin-like growth factor I receptor gene expression. *Mol Cell Biol* 1995;15: 3516-3522.

[86] Waffarn, F; Davis, EP. Effects of antenatal corticosteroids on the hypothalamic-pituitary-adrenocortical axis of the fetus and newborn: experimental findings and clinical considerations. *Am J Obstet Gynecol* 2012;207(6): 446-454.

[87] Patel, R; Patel, M; Tsai, R; et al. LXRβ is required for glucocorticoid-induced hyperglycemia and hepatosteatosis in mice. *J Clin Invest* 2011;121: 431-441.

[88] White, PC; Speiser, PW. Congenital Adrenal Hyperplasia due to 21-Hydroxylase Deficiency. *Endocr Rev* 2000;21: 245-291.

[89] Miles, HL; Gidlöf, S; Nordenström, A; Ong, KK; Hughes, IA. The role of androgens in fetal growth: observational study in two genetic models of disordered androgen signalling. *Arch Dis Child Fetal Neonatal Ed* 2010;95: F435-438.

[90] Charmandari, E; Kino, T; Ichijo, T; Chrousos, GP. Generalized glucocorticoid resistance: clinical aspects, molecular mechanisms, and implications of a rare genetic disorder. *J Clin Endocrinol Metab* 2008;93: 1563-1572.

[91] Mendonca, BB; Leite, MV; de Castro, M; et al. Female Pseudohermaphroditism Caused by a Novel Homozygous Missense Mutation of the GR Gene. *J Clin Endocrinol Metab* 2002;87: 1805-1809.

[92] White, PC. Ontogeny of adrenal steroid biosynthesis: why girls will be girls. *J Clin Invest* 2006;116: 872-874.

[93] Mesiano, S; Jaffe, RB. Developmental and functional biology of the primate fetal adrenal cortex. *Endocr Rev* 1997;18: 378-403.

In: Macrosomia and Birth Weight
Editor: Larry P. Harris

ISBN: 978-1-63483-124-6

Chapter III

Determinants and Outcomes of Macrosomia in a Mediterranean Island Population

C. Savona-Ventura*[*] *and J. Craus
Department of Obstetrics and Gynaecology,
University of Malta Medical School, Malta

Abstract

Infant birth weight is known to be dependent on the interplay of nature and nurture. An excessive birth weight has been associated with definite socio-biological maternal characteristics which in part contribute to the genetic makeup of the child and to determining the degree of nutritional capacity made available to the child during intrauterine existence. Macrosomic infants are more likely to be born to relatively older multiparous mothers who are obese and potentially diabetic exhibiting excessive weight gain during pregnancy – all features promoting abundant nutrient availability during intrauterine life. The excessive birth weight of the infant further poses increased perinatal risks to both the mother and child increasing the likelihood for intrapartum

[*] Corresponding author: Prof. C. Savona-Ventura MD DScMed, Department of Obstetrics and Gynaecology, University of Malta Medical School, Mater Dei Hospital, Msida, Malta. E-mail address: charles.savona-ventura@um.edu.mt.

problems including prolonged labour and foetal anoxia, an increased risk for operative delivery with the related maternal and infant morbidity, and risks for shoulder dystocia. Besides the short-term problems to the infant posed by the prolonged labour and intrapartum trauma, macrosomia is also associated with long-term metabolic consequences for the child with a greater predisposition to childhood adiposity and adulthood carbohydrate intolerance.

Introduction

The eventual body weight at birth of the infant has been shown to be dependent upon the interplay of different factors that include foetal factors such as gender, the genetic makeup of the parents determining stature, and the degree of nutrition made available to the developing foetus. Many of these factors have long been accepted determinants of foetal size at birth. A 19th century textbook identified the intrauterine growth determining factors to include (1) the gender of the child; (2) the parity of the mother; (3) maternal age; and (4) parental constitution [1]. The role of intrauterine nutrition and the relationship of diabetes in determining foetal birth weight was originally identified in the 1920s but was formalized by Jørgen Pedersen in 1967 who formulated the hypothesis concerning how the foetus is affected by maternal hyperglycemia – now known as the "Pedersen Hypothesis" [2].

Macrosomia (from the Greek *macro* = large; *sōma* = body) generally refers to infants with a birth weight of 4000 g or more. A better alternative definition to identify infants at outcome risk is to consider macrosomic infants to be "large for gestational age" (LGA) basing the cut-off birth weight to a value above the 90th percentile for that gestational age. It has however been suggested that macrosomia should be considered significant if the birth weight is 4500 g or more, and LGA if the birth weight is greater than the 97th percentile or two standard deviations above the mean. The latter cut-off points identify more accurately those infants with a greater risk of perinatal and long-term morbidity and mortality.

Study Population Characteristics

The Maltese Archipelago situated in the central Mediterranean is made up of three inhabitable islands that together make up only 316 km^2. With a population of 417,432 individuals in 2011, the islands are by far the most densely populated European Union Member State with an average of 1,325 persons per km^2 [3]. The overall health of the population is consistent with that of a developed country with a life expectancy of 83.1 years in females and 78.9 years in males. The crude birth rate in 2011 stood at 10.3 per 1000 population while the crude death rate stands at 7.9 per 1000 population [4]. Dietary changes associated with the high standard of living have contributed to making the metabolic syndrome and its comorbidities the primary health problem of the population. Rates of the comorbidities of the metabolic syndrome are particularly high in the adult Maltese population – adiposity with a BMI $\geq$25 kg/m^2 accounts for 76.8% in men and 54.9% in women; hyperglycaemia of $\geq$7.0 mmol/l: men 9.0%, women 10.7%; hypercholesterolaemia: men 68.8%, women 56.1%; hypertension: men 33.1%, women 31.4%. Long-term complications of these conditions, such as heart disease and stroke account for 38.3% of all deaths [5, 6].

The presence of metabolic syndrome features including maternal adiposity and gestational hyperglycaemia-diabetes contributes towards a state of hypernutrition of the developing foetus predisposing to elevated birth weights. It appears that the rates of both maternal adiposity and gestational hyperglycaemia-diabetes have increased over the decades. Cross-sectional studies conducted on Maltese population in 1983 and 2010 suggest an increase in the mean third trimester body mass index of Maltese pregnant women from 27.9 $\pm$ 5.5 to 29.9 $\pm$ 6.2 kg/m^2. There has also be an accompanying apparent increase in the prevalence of gestational hyperglycaemia-diabetes based on the WHO 1983 diagnostic criteria from 11.5% to 15.5%. The latter rate actually translates to 16.5% of the whole pregnant population using the newly proposed IADPSG diagnostic criteria [7, 8].

In spite of the apparent increase in two contributing confounders, there has been an apparent drop in mean birth rates throughout the decades. The mean birth weight in 2009 stood at 3252 $\pm$ 516 gm. There appears to have been a statistically significant decreasing trend in the mean birth weights of infants born over the last fifty years from a mean of 3338 $\pm$ 469 gm in 1965 [Figure 1] [9]. The proportion of infants born with a birth weight of 4000 gm or greater has similarly been shown to have decreased from 18.4% in the 1950s to 10.2% in 1981 and further to 4.4% in 2009 [10]. The reasons for this fall may be due to better management of hyperglycaemic states and earlier recourse to delivery in these cases potentially leaving these infants LGA but not necessarily macrosomic on the basis of eventual birth weight.

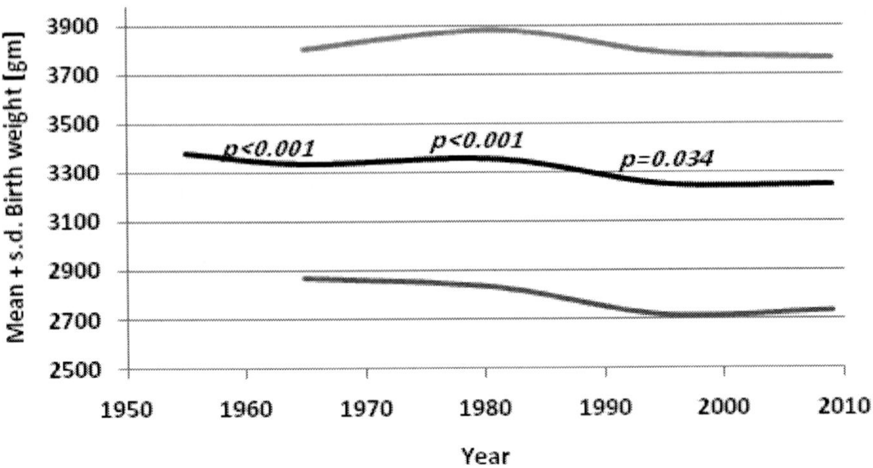

Figure 1. Mean + 1 s.d. birth weight – Maltese population 1951-59, 1965, 1981, 1995, 2009; Statistical significant: t-test comparing with 2009.

Parental Contributors

Genetic determinants certainly contribute towards the tendency for infants to be large for gestational age. Epidemiological studies have suggested that genetic factors may actually account for 30-80% of the variance in birth weight [11]. A familial trend has been noted in a Scandinavian population between parental and infant birth weights. However, the authors found parental birth weight to be a rather poor predictor accounting for only about 5.6% of the variation in infant birth weight [12]. Similarly, a study carried out in Norway assessing parental-offspring covariances in birth weight showed that height and weight of both parents were associated with variation in birth weight, though parental variables could only explain 10% of the variation in mean offspring birth weight [13].

In the Maltese population, the mean birth weight of the infant increased progressively with increasing maternal height from a mean birth weight of 3062 ± 516 g in women with a height less than 150 cm to 3421 ± 518 g in those women with a height of 170 cm or more [Figure 2] [14]. A similar interrelationship was noted in the mean birth weight which became higher with increasing maternal BMI with a mean birth weight of 3066 ± 496 g in women with a BMI < 20 kg/m^2 increasing to a mean birth weight of 3340 ± 552 g in women with a BMI of ≥ 30 kg/m^2 [Figure 2] [14]. The proportion of macrosomic infants similarly increased progressively with increasing maternal BMI increasing from 1.9% in lean women with a BMI of < 20 kg/m^2 to 3.9% in those with a BMI of 20-24, to 6.8% in those with a BMI of 25-29, and 9.5% in women with a BMI of 30 kg/m^2 or more [15].

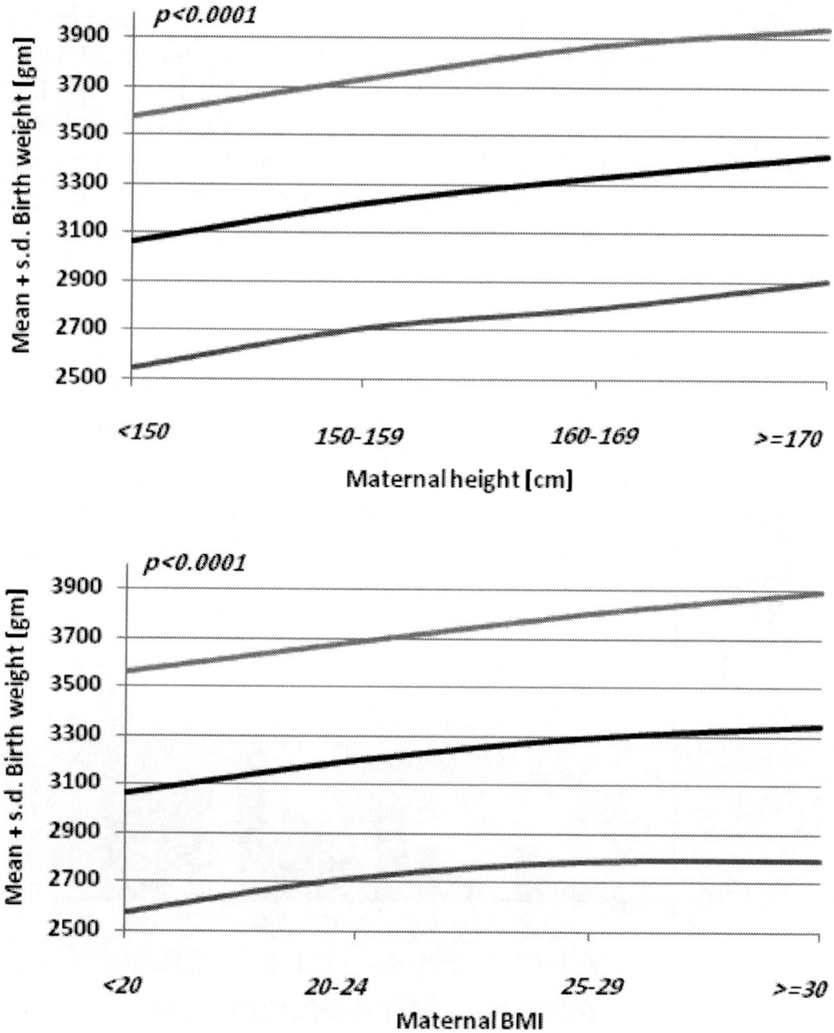

Figure 2. Mean + 1 s.d. birth weight by maternal height and BMI – Maltese population 1999-2006.

The influence of maternal stature on the infant birth weight is probably a reflection of genetic determinants; however the influence of maternal BMI more probably reflects the increased availability of nutrients being presented to the child during intrauterine life. A relationship between a higher incidence of macrosomia and increasing weight gain during pregnancy irrespective of maternal BMI has been similarly demonstrated in the Maltese population [Figure 3]. A macrosomia rate greater than 10% was associated with an antenatal weight gain of 15 kg or more in women with a BMI 25-29 kg/m^2, and with a weight gain of 10 kg or more in women with a BMI >30 kg/m^2. Women with a BMI < 25 kg/m^2 showed a macrosomia rate of under 10% irrespective of the degree of weight gain during pregnancy. Conversely low weight gain during pregnancy especially in the lean woman was inversely related to the development of macrosomia [15, 16].

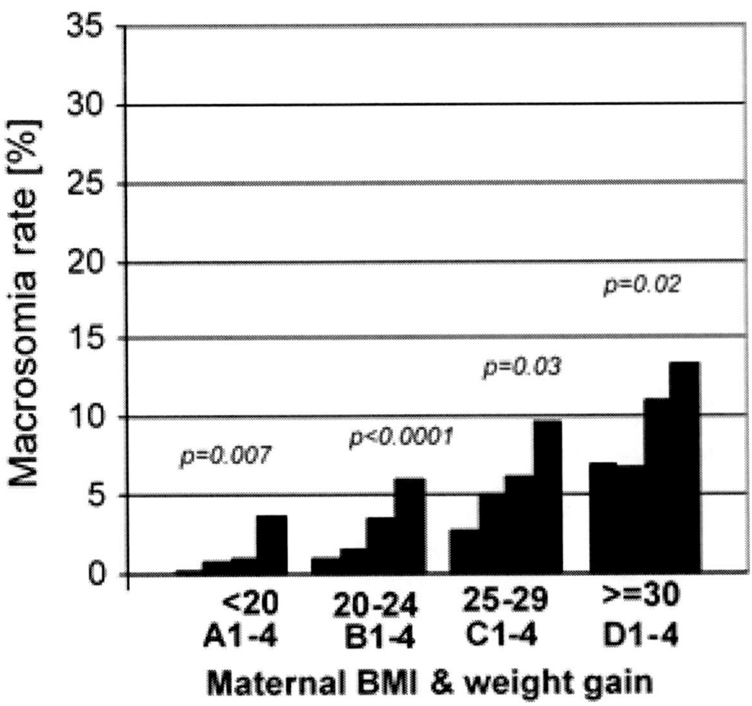

Figure 3. Macrosomia rate by maternal BMI and weight gain during pregnancy; *Weight gain during pregnancy: 1 = 0-4; 2 = 5-9; 3 = 10-14; 4 = >15 kg.*

The relationship between overeating and excessive birth weight was first proposed by Hugo Ehrenfest in 1919 [17]. Epidemiological studies have further shown that a high birth weight is related not simply to the glycaemic status of the mother during pregnancy but also relates to the mother body mass and weight gain during pregnancy irrespective of the carbohydrate metabolism status of the woman [18]. Transgenerational studies in animal models have linked the predisposition to macrosomia to a number of different mechanisms involving foetal pancreatic and hypothalamic development. Second and third generation pups of STZ-injected diabetic rats developed pancreatic islet cell hyperplasia and beta cell generation when exposed to a hypernutritional state during intrauterine life. The hyperplasia increased the endocrine tissue volume density but seemingly decreased the density of the granulated beta cells volume [19]. Similar pancreatic alterations have been noted in foetuses of diabetic human mothers [20], the severity being apparently related to the degree of maternal glycaemia and body mass index [21]. Other processes influencing foetuses born to diabetic mothers include the malprogramming of hypothalamic orexigenic and anorexigenic neurons, possibly mediated through a raised foetal and neonatal leptin [22].

The hypothesis of the mechanism whereby maternal hyperglycaemia contributed to excessive foetal growth and the predisposition to macrosomia was formulated by Jørgen Pedersen in 1967 [2]. Pedersen Hypothesis maintains that hyperglycemia in the mother results in a relative hyperglycaemia in the foetus which in turn stimulates the foetal pancreas to produce excess insulin. The resulting hyperinsulinaemia produces interalia adiposity and macrosomia [Figure 4] [23]. In the Maltese population, the rate of macrosomia increased progressively from 5.8% in non-diabetics to 12.2% in women with gestational diabetes (Risk Ratio 2.10; $p < 0.0001$) and 22.8% in women with pre-existing diabetes mellitus (RR 3.93; $p < 0.0001$) [24].

Other maternal characteristics shown to contribute towards a greater predisposition of macrosomia in this population include maternal age of 30 years or more (RR 1.38; $p < 0.0001$), previous parity (RR 1.55; $p < 0.0001$), or previous miscarriage (RR 1.20; $p = 0.04$). The presence of hypertensive disease was inversely related to the macrosomia risk (RR 0.72; $p = 0.02$). There did not appear to be any statistical relationships between a history of antepartum haemorrhage and the necessity for ovulation induction intervention to achieve a pregnancy [24]. The relationship of these maternal characteristics may be indirect correlates to intrauterine nutrition with advanced age and parity being related to a greater risk of hyperglycaemia and overnutrition; while the inverse relationship with hypertensive disease was an indirect correlate to undernutrition caused by placental insufficiency.

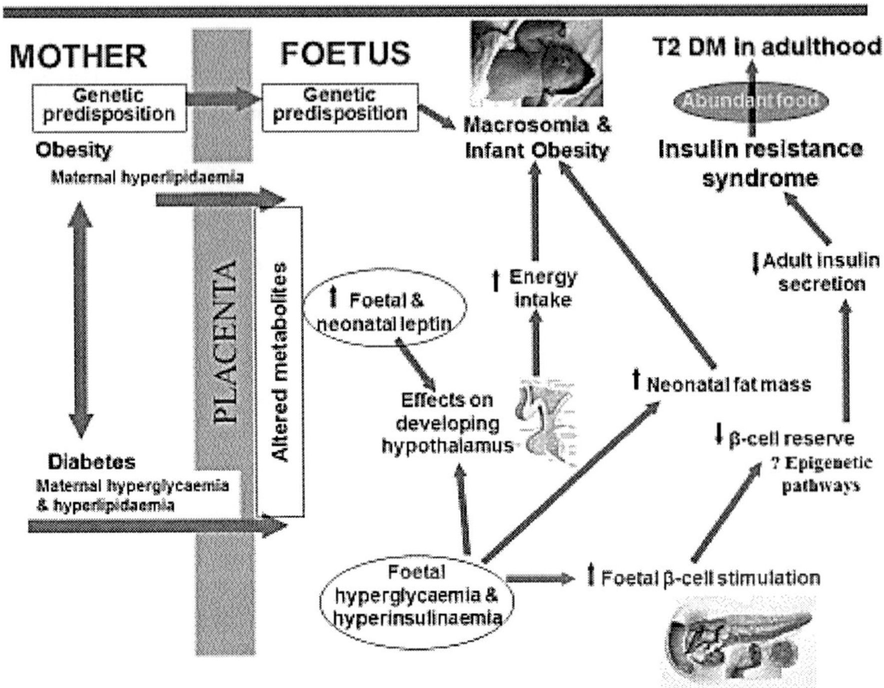

Figure 4. Modified Pedersen Hypothesis.

Foetal Contributors

Birth weight means for Maltese new-borns during the period 1995-2009 confirm that male infants birth weight means exceeded those of female infants at all gestations [Table 1]. At 40 weeks of gestation, there was a statistically significant difference of 125 gm between the sexes [9]. Macrosomic infants were statistically (RR 1.64; $p < 0.0001$) more likely to be male rather than female [24].

Animal and human studies have suggested that the genetic makeup of the developing foetus may be involved in fetal growth. In the mouse model, gene knockout studies have confirmed the relationship between normal foetal growth and insulin-related genes such as insulin-like growth factor (IGF)-I, IGF-II, IGF receptor type 1, insulin, insulin receptor, and insulin receptor substrate [11, 25, 26]. In humans, a 200 gram birth weight increase was found to be associated the homozygous presence of the insulin variable number tandem repeat class III genotype. Besides weight, the genotype also influenced length and head circumference [27]. Specific genetic disorder caused by errors in genomic imprinting, such as Beckwith-Wiedemann syndrome (chromosome 11p15 rearrangements), Sotos syndrome (mutations of NSD1 gene), Periman syndrome (disorder of 2q37.2 on chromosome 2 – DIS3L2 gene) and MOMO syndrone (disruption of 20p11.23 – LINC00237 gene), have been directly associated with the development of macrosomia in the infant. These conditions however are relatively rare genetic conditions that play a minimal role in the aetiology of macrosomia [28, 29, 30, 31]. Other conditions contributing to later childhood syndromatic adiposity, such as Down's syndrome (Trisomy 21) which acts by altering the production of obesity-related hormones, may not be associated with macrosomia at birth. The mean Maltese birth weight of Trisomy 21 infants born at term gestation during 1999-2006 was statistically lower than the mean birth weight of normal Maltese term infants (2900.8 $\pm$ 600.5 gm n = 43 vs 3305.9 $\pm$ 434.2 gm n = 28147; $p < 0.0001$).

Table 1. Birth weight centiles by gender and gestation – Maltese population 1995-2009

Gestation [weeks]	Male Birth weight [gm]		Female Birth weight [gm]	
	50th centile	91st centile	50th centile	91st centile
42	3603	4193	3469	4030
41	3525	4100	3392	3943
40	3431	3995	3301	3845
39	3308	3877	3180	3733
38	3159	3758	3033	3621
37	2986	3631	2862	3502
36	2793	3484	2671	3363
35	2590	3315	2468	3203
34	2381	3125	2260	3019
33	2171	2914	2052	2812
32	1964	2683	1849	2585
31	1764	2436	1654	2345
30	1572	2180	1471	2099

Consequences of Macrosomia

Infant size has traditionally been shown to be associated with significant effects on the intrapartum outcome. In Maltese obstetric practice, macrosomic infants were more likely to require an operative intervention in the form of an emergency Caesarean section (RR 1.32; $p < 0.0001$) or an operative vaginal delivery (RR 1.54, $p < 0.0001$). There was no difference in the relative risk for macrosomic babies to require an elective operative abdominal delivery. Because of the increased use of Caesarean section for macrosomic infants, delivery trauma did not show any statistical increase with increasing birth weight. The second stage of labour appeared to be increasingly complicated in the presence of macrosomic infants with an increasing predisposition towards shoulder dystocia (RR 6.75; $P < 0.0001$) in spite of the increasing use of Caesarean section. The increased Caesarean section rate in the presence of macrosomic infants in current obstetric practice significantly reduced the risks of intrapartum trauma so that the perinatal outcome did not appear to be adversely influenced by infant birth weight showing no statistical differences in the rates of low Apgar scores at 5 minutes and perinatal deaths. None of the infants suffered from respiratory distress, seizures or significant hyperbilirubinaemia in the perinatal period. Infant feeding appeared to be statistically dependent on infant body weight, so that proportionately more macrosomic infants were fully breastfed at the time of discharge from hospital (RR 1.24; $p = 0.0009$). However, infants weighing ≥4500 gm were more likely to require artificial feeding as a primary form of feeding or as an adjuvant so that while 44.4% of infants with a birth weight of 4000-4499 g were solely breastfed, only 25.8% of infants with a birth weight of ≥4500 g were solely breastfed. Women delivering excessive high birth weight infants ≥4500 g vaginally also appeared to have a higher rate of problems with the delivery of the placenta so that while surgical evacuation of the placenta was required in 0.8% of pregnancies delivering infants weight 4000-4499 g, the rate of retained placenta was 1.6% in those pregnancies delivering infants weighing ≥4500 g [24].

The intrauterine over-nutrition predisposing to macrosomia also sets a series of adaptive mechanism that have long-term consequences on the health of the child. In the Maltese context, macrosomic infants have been shown to have a greater risk of developing childhood adiposity at five and nine years of life [Figure 5]. Maltese macrosomic-born infants were more likely to be overweight or obese at 5-years of age when compared to their normal birth weight counterparts (92.0% vs 19.4%; $p < 0.0001$). The body parameters reflecting adiposity of these children were also elevated though the differences did not reach statistical significance (mean BMI 17.5 ± 2.7 vs 16.7 ± 2.2 kg/m^2 – mean body weight 22.7 ± 4.8 vs 20.8 ± 3.7 kg – mean waist circumference 55.5 ± 5.4 vs 54.7 ± 7.0 cm). There was no difference in mean body height. Similar observations were made at 9-years of age. Macrosomic-born Maltese 9-year olds were therefore statistically more likely to be overweight or obese than their normal birth weight counterparts (77.8% vs 30.6%; $p < 0.0001$) with higher mean BMI values (22.5 ± 4.7 vs 19.2 ± 4.0 kg/m^2; $p = 0.002$), mean body weight (42.0 ± 9.0 vs 35.2 ± 9.2 kg; $p = 0.004$), and mean waist circumference (71.6 ± 8.1 vs 64.6 ± 10.9 cm; $p = 0.01$). The macrosomic-born 9-year old children also showed a statistically higher mean body height (1.4 ± 0.1 vs 1.3 ± 0.1 m; $p = 0.0001$) [32].

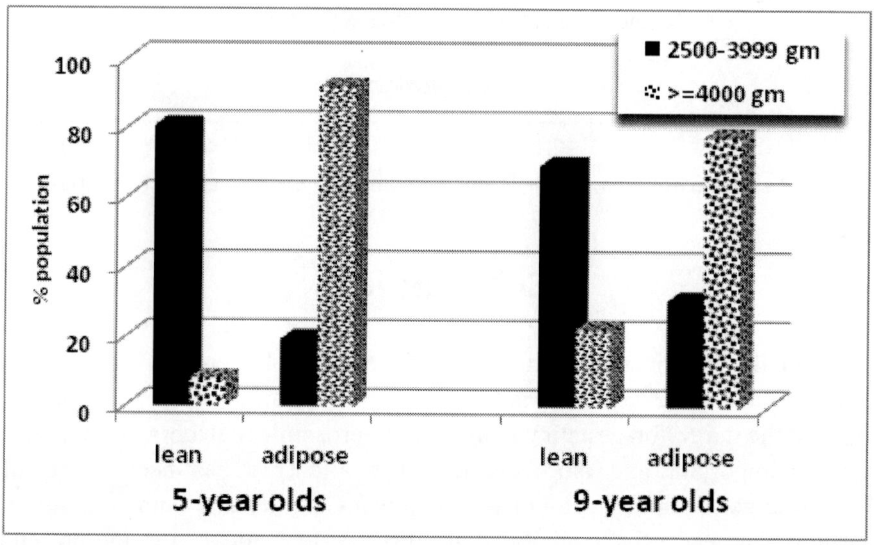

Figure 5. Proportion of adiposity in Macrosomic-born and normal birth weight Maltese infants at 5 and 9 years of life.

The female macrosomic infants born with birth weight of > = 4500 gm have also been shown to have a higher predisposition to develop adult-onset gestational diabetes (RR 2.73). The risk ratio for developing GDM in women born with birth weight ranges of 2500-3999 and 4000-4499 gm were 0.98 and 0.62 respectively [33].

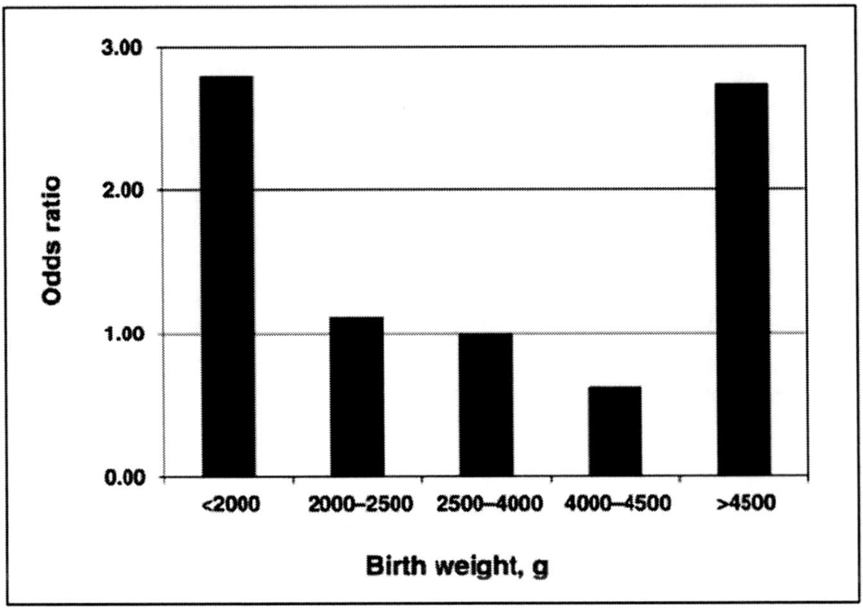

Figure 6. Risk Ratio of developing GDM by birth weight – Maltese women [p = 0.005].

Conclusion

Animal experimental studies and epidemiological evidence have suggested that genetic predispositions may play a minor role in contributing towards the large-for-gestational age or macrosomic newborn. However, a definate important and more significant relationship has been repeatedly shown between the development of the LGA neonate and intrauterine nutrition. The excessive availabilty of nutrients, as evidenced in the presence of maternal adiposity, excessive weight gain in pregnancy, or hyperglycaemia caused by the diabetic syndromes, contribute significantly towards foetal adiposity. The hypernutritional state of the developing foetus generates structural and functional changes that make the individual more susceptible to developing childhood and adulthood adiposity later on in life with all the attendant co-morbidities and associated risks for premature death. It is ironical that the present generation of children, because of a significant improvement in the socio-economic and nutrient availability, may actually be at a higher risk of a premature death when compared to their parents. The LGA neonate also is at risk during the intrapartum and early neonatal period being more susceptible to intrapartum trauma and adverse biochemical alterations.

These observations present important chances and challenges of adipose-preventive medicine. Prevention of macrosomia, and consequently reducing the tendency to child and adult adiposity, should follow early identification of at-risk pregnany women and the introduction of timely intervention with healthy lifestyle patterns and pharmacological control. Pregnant women at risk of having a macrosomic infant – such as those suffering from diabetes mellitus, the adipose woman, or those exhibiting excessive weight gains during pregnancy – should receive targeted dietary advice and close metabolic follow-up throughout their pregnancy. This will ensure that the developing foetus will be presented with as optimum a physiology as possible maintaining euglycemia and normal insulin levels throughout the pregnancy. The nutritional advice needs to be further supplemented by a realistic physical exercise program. These lifestyle interventions should ideally start pre-conceptionally aiming at weight reduction before embarking on a pregnancy and maintained right through pregnancy. The LGA infant should be considered as having a life-long increased risk for developing features of the metabolic syndrome. Parents, particularly mothers, of LGA children should be encouraged to adopt and maintain healthy nutrition patterns for the whole family. In addition, early involvement and encouragement to participate in sport activities of the macrosomic-born child may hopefully result in regular physical exercise which helps to counter the inherent tendency towards developing adiposity. An effective life-long intervention programme needs to involve multidisciplinary teams at every intervention point thus ensuring with regular follow-up that both the child and the parents are subject to repeated attempts at re-enforcing healthy lifestyle intervention. This requires a serious commitment by health service providers. However even with the best of resource provision convincing individuals to maintain a life-long health lifestyle is not simple or easy process. Only a minority will be successful, the majority will be successful in adopting a healthy behaviour for themselves and/or their children for a short duration or none at all. Any intervention programme requiring long-term adherence must utilize the principles of psychotherapeutic Cognitive Behavioural Therapy (CBT) which attempts to promote a sense of self-efficacy accepting the condition and discovering adaptive coping skills for themselves thus empowering the individual to fully understand the problem and adopt a plan of action to achieve self-identified reasonable goals and targets [34].

References

[1] Spiegelber O. A text book of midwifery. London: *New Sydenham Soc.*, 1887, 2 vols; 1: 123.

[2] Pedersen J. The Pregnant diabetic and her Newborn: Problems and management. *Baltimore: Williams & Wilkins Co.*, 1967.

[3] N.S.O. Census of population and housing 2011 – Final Report. *Malta: National Statistics Office,* 2014.

[4] N.S.O. Malta in Figures 2012. *Malta: National Statistics Office,* 2012.

[5] N.S.O. Demographic Review 2010. *Malta: National Statistics Office,* 2011.

[6] D.H.I.R. The European Health Examination Survey – Pilot Study 2010. Malta: *Directorate for Health Information and research,* 2012.

[7] Savona-Ventura C, Schranz AG, Chazan B. The clinical significance of gestational impaired glucose tolerance in the Maltese population. *Arch Perinatal Med,* 1997; 3: 55-64.

[8] Craus J, Savona-Ventura C, Vassallo J. Prevalence of GDM in the Maltese population. Twelfth Meeting of the Mediterranean Group for the Study of Diabetes April 28 – May 1, 2011. *Morocco: MGSD,* 2011, pp.159.

[9] Zammit V, Zammit P, Savona-Ventura C, Buhagiar A, Grech V. Maltese national birth weight for gestational age centile values. *Malta Med J,* 2010; 22(2): 19-24.

[10] Savona-Ventura C, Savona-Ventura S. Endogenous physiological teratogenesis. The Maltese population – A Case Study. Germany: *Lambert Academic publ.,* 2013.

[11] Johnston LB, Clark AJL, Savage MO. Genetic factors contributing to birth weight. *Arch Dis Child Fetal Neonatal Ed,* 2002; 86: F2-F3.

[12] Langhoff-Roos J, Lindmark G, Gustavson KH, et al. Relative effect of parental birth weight on infant birth weight at term. *Clin Genet,* 1987; 32: 240–248.

[13] P. Magnus, K. Berg, T. Bjerkedal, W. E. Nance. Parental determinants of birth weight. *Clinical Genetics,* 1984; 26(5): 397-405.

[14] Savona-Ventura C, Buttigieg GG, Grima S, Vella M. Anthropomorphic characteristics as obstetric risk determinants. *Int J Risk Saf Med,* 2008; 20(3): 155-160.

[15] Savona-Ventura C, Grima S, Vella K. Maternal BMI and antenatal weight gain as determinants of obstetric outcome. *Int J Diabetes & Metabolism,* 2008a; 16: 51-53.

[16] Savona-Ventura C, Buttigieg GG, Mifsud M. Maternal weight gain and fetal growth. *Malta Med J* 2009; 21(2): 22-25.

[17] Luke B, Keith L. Principles and practice of maternal nutrition. USA: *Parthenon Publishing Group*, 1992.

[18] Catalano PM, Hauquel-De Mouzon S. Is it time to revisit the Pedersen hypothesis in the face of the obesity epidemic? *Am J Obstet Gynecol,* 2011; 204: 479-487.

[19] Aerts L, Van Assche FA. Is gestational diabetes an acquired condition? *J Develop Physio,* 1979; 1: 219-225.

[20] Van Assche FA, Gepts W, Aerts L. The fetal endocrine pancreas in diabetes (human). *Diabetologia*, 1976; 12: 423.

[21] Hultquist GT & Olding L. Pancreatic islet fibrosis in young infants of diabetic mothers. *Lancet,* 1975; ii: 1015-1016.

[22] Franke K, Harder T, Aerts L, Melchior K, Fahrenkrog S, Rodekamp E, Ziska T, Van Assche FA, Dudenhausen JW & Plagemann A. Programming of orexigenic and anorexigenic hypothalamic neurons in offspring of treated and untreated diabetic mother rats. *Brain Res,* 2005; 1031(2): 276-283.

[23] Pedersen J. Weight and length at birth of infants of diabetic mothers. *Acta Endocrinol,* 1954;16: 330-342.

[24] Savona-Ventura C, Chircop M. Determinants for macrosomia in a Mediterranean island community. *Int J Diabetes & Metabolism*, 2004; 12(3): 44-48.

[25] Accili D, Nakae J, Kim JJ, et al. Targeted gene mutations define the roles of insulin and IGF-I receptors in mouse embryonic development. *J Pediatr Endocrinol Metab,* 1999; 12: 475–485.

[26] Baker J, Liu JP, Robertson EJ, et al. Role of insulin-like growth factors in embryonic and postnatal growth. Role of insulin-like growth factors in embryonic and postnatal growth. *Cell,* 1993;75: 73–82.

[27] Dunger DB, Ong KK, Huxtable SJ, et al. Association of the INS VNTR with size at birth. ALSPAC Study Team. Avon Longitudinal Study of Pregnancy and Childhood. *Nat Genet,* 1998; 19: 98–100.

[28] Wiedemann HR. Familial malformation complex with umbilical hernia and macroglossia - a "new syndrome"?. *Journal de génétique humaine,* 1964; 13: 223–232.

[29] Kurotaki, N; Imaizumi, K; Harada, N; Masuno, M; Kondoh, T; Nagai, T; Ohashi, H; Naritomi, K; Tsukahara, M; Makita, Y; Sugimoto, T; Sonoda, T; Hasegawa, T; Chinen, Y; Tomita Ha, H. A.; Kinoshita, A; Mizuguchi, T; Yoshiura Ki, K; Ohta, T; Kishino, T; Fukushima, Y; Niikawa, N; Matsumoto, N. Haploinsufficiency of NSD1 causes Sotos syndrome. *Nature Genetics,* 2002; 30 (4): 365–6.

[30] Perlman M. Perlman syndrome: familial renal dysplasia with Wilms tumor, fetal gigantism, and multiple congenital anomalies. *Am J Med Genet*, 1986; 25 (Pt 4): 793–795.

[31] Vu PY1, Toutain J, Cappellen D, Delrue MA, Daoud H, El Moneim AA, Barat P, Montaubin O, Bonnet F, Dai ZQ, Philippe C, Tran CT, Rooryck C, Arveiler B, Saura R, Briault S, Lacombe D, Taine L. A homozygous balanced reciprocal translocation suggests LINC00237 as a candidate gene for MOMO (macrosomia, obesity, macrocephaly, and ocular abnormalities) syndrome. *Am J Med Genet A*, 2012; 158A (11): 2849-2856.

[32] Scerri C, Savona-Ventura C. Early metabolic imprinting as a determinant of childhood obesity. *International J Diabetes Mellitus,* 2010; 2: 175-178.

[33] Savona-Ventura C, Chircop M. Birth weight influence on the subsequent development of gestational diabetes mellitus. *Acta Diabetologica,* 2003; 40: 101-104.

[34] Sage N, Sowden M, Chorlton E, Edeleanu A. CBT for Chronic illness and Palliative Care – a Workbook and Toolkit. *England: John Wiley & Sons Ltd;* 2008.

In: Macrosomia and Birth Weight
Editor: Larry P. Harris

ISBN: 978-1-63483-124-6

Chapter IV

The Effect of Cigarette Smoking on Birth Weight and Placental Weight: A Study in Two Italian Populations

Fulvia Gloria-Bottini * ***and Egidio Bottini***
Department of Biomedicine and Prevention, University of TorVergata, Rome, Italy

Abstract

Objective: The effect of cigarette smoking on the ratio of Placenta Weight vs Birth Weight (PW/BW) is influenced by many factors. We have compared the effect of cigarette smoking on BW and PW in two Italian populations living in different environments.

Methods: We have studied 384 newborn infants from the White population of Rome and 404 newborn infants from the population of Penne. In the metropolitan area of Rome the environmental pollution is high while the rural population of Penne lives in a pure environment.

* Corresponding author: Fulvia Gloria-Bottini, MD, Department of Biomedicine and Prevention, University of Tor Vergata, Via Monpellier, 100133 Rome, Italy, Phone: +39 0630889514 Email: gloria@med.uniroma2.it.

Results: The negative effect of smoking on BW is much stronger in Rome than in Penne. No effect on PW is present in Penne and only a slight not statistically significant effect in Rome. In young women there is a less marked effect of smoking on BW. No differences is observed between sexes.

Conclusion: Besides confirming previous observations on the greater effect of maternal smoking on BW as compared to PW, the data suggest that environmental pollution may enhance the effect of smoking. A cumulative action of toxic substances of cigarette smoking on the reproductive apparatus may result in a more evident effect of smoking on intrauterine development in older women.

Keywords: Cigarette smoking; birth weight; placental weight; BW/PW ratio; environmental pollution; maternal age

Introduction

The association between maternal cigarette smoking and low birth weight (BW) is well established [1-7], the ratio placental weight (PW) to BW is influenced by maternal cigarette smoking resulting in a high PW/BW ratio in smoking mothers [8]. This ratio is an independent risk factor for cardiovascular diseases in adulthood and the problem of the effect of smoking on this parameter has been considered in several studies and more recently in a large cohort of Tasmanian newborns [9-14].

We hypothesized that environmental factors amplify the negative effects of smoking during pregnancy on placental weight and fetal birth weight and in the present paper we report a study on two Italian populations living in different environments. We have examined the effect of environment, maternal age and newborn sex on the association of maternal smoking with BW and PW.

Material and Methods

We have studied 384 consecutive newborn infants from the White population of Rome (collected in the Department of Obstetrics and Gynecology of Rome University) and 404 consecutive newborn infants from the population of Penne (collected in the Department of Obstetrics and

Gynecology of S. Massimo Hospital). In the population of Rome newborn infants only were studied, while in the population of Penne the mothers also were studied. The population of Rome is a mixture of people coming from all Italian regions: in this metropolitan area the environmental pollution is high and winters are relatively mild (mean winter temperature 12°C, mean summer temperature 30°C). The population of Penne is homogeneous and the people are descendants of an old italic populations called "Vestini." This rural population lives in a pure environment and winters are cold (mean winter temperature 4°C, mean summer temperature 28°C). In Rome during the year 2013 the limit of 50 μg of fine particulate air pollution was exceeded in 41 days... In Penne such measurements have not been performed: indeed the urban center is very small and the traffic is not comparable to that of Rome. The percent proportion of smoking mothers is 37.8% in Rome and 9.2% in Penne.

Verbal informed consent was obtained from the mothers to participate to the study. The data were collected few decades ago from medical records. Ethical Committee was not established and the study was approved by the Department of Pediatrics.

Statistical analyses were carried by commercial software (SPSS). Because of random missing of data on some variables the number of subjects are not the same for BW and PW. This is particularly evident in the data from Penne.

Results

Table 1 shows some characteristics of the samples studied.

Table 2 shows the distribution of neonatal BW and PW in relation to maternal smoking in the populations of Penne and Rome. The negative effect of smoking on BW is much stronger in Rome than in Penne: 200 gr in Rome vs 100 gr in Penne. No effect of smoking on PW is present in Penne and only a slight not statistically significant effect is observed in Rome.

Table 3 shows the role of maternal age on the effect of cigarette smoking on BW and PW.

In both Rome and Penne the effect on BW is much less marked in puerperae aging 27 years (median value of age distribution) or less as compared to that observed in puerperae aging more than 27 years. No appreciable difference in relation to maternal age is observed for PW.

No appreciable difference is observed between males and females (data not shown).

Table 1. Characteristics of the samples studied

	Rome		Penne	
	Mean	**S.E.**	**Mean**	**S.E.**
Maternal Age (yrs)	28.50	0.31	27.15	0.26
N° abortions	1.22	0.02	0.14	0.03
N° of pregnancies	2.08	0.07	1.68	0.07
Gestational age (wks)	39.77	0.09	39.66	0.06
N° of cigarettes/day	6.71	0.06	7.01	0.11
% Proportion of newborn Homozygote				
AB0	48.0%		46.1%	
PGM_1	50.0%		47.4%	
ACP_1	54.7%		52.8%	

[a] S.E. = Standard Error.
[b] AB0 = Proportion of 0 blood group.
[c] PGM_1 = Phospho Gluco Mutase locus 1.
[d] ACP_1 = Acid Phosphatase locus 1.
[e] The number of cigarettes/day had been not registered for all women. The mean refers to the women in whom the number of cigarettes had been registered.

Table 2. Distribution of birth weight and placental weight in relation to smoking

	Penne			Rome		
	Mean	**S.E.**	**N°**	**Mean**	**S.E.**	**N°**
Birth Weight (gr)						
Smoking	3262	77.7	37	3169	44.6	145
Non smoking	3360	23.2	367	3383	31.4	239
Student-t Mann-Whitney	T=1.263	p=0.206		T=4.022	p=0.000 P=0.000	
Placental Weight (gr)						
Smoking	596	23.0	22	563	10.8	138
Non smoking	595	8.3	270	584	8.7	225
Student-t	T=0.004	p=0.996		T=1.441	p=0.151	

[a] S.E. = Standard Error.

Table 3. Distribution of birth weight and placental weight in relation to maternal age and smoking

		Penne			Rome		
		Mean	**S.E.**	**N°**	**Mean**	**S.E.**	**N°**
		Birth weight (gr)					
Maternal age ≤27 yrs	Smoking	3381	98.3	22	3214	59.0	71
	Non smoking	3327	25.1	195	3383	43.1	106
	Student-t Mann-Whitney	T=0.656 p=0.512			T=2.434 p=0.016 P=0.037		
		Placental weight (gr)					
	Smoking	627	37.6	14	564	14.6	71
	Non smoking	586	10.4	105	583	8.7	106
	Student-t	T=0.909	p=0.365		T=1.248	p=0.214	
Maternal age >27 yrs		**Birth weight (gr)**					
	Smoking	3113	121.6	14	3110	69.7	74
	Non smoking	3.403	42.4	147	3379	44.9	133
	Student-t Mann-Whitney	T=2.032	p=0.044 P=0.017		T=3.330	p=0.001 P=0.002	
		Placental weight (gr)					
	Smoking	540	37.0	7	561	16.7	74
	Non smoking	589	13.7	105	581	13.2	133
	Student-t	T=0.956	p=0.341		T=0.900	p=0.369	

[a] S.E. = Standard Error.

Discussion

The present data confirm the increase of PW/BW ratio in smoking mothers and suggest that environmental conditions and maternal age influence the effect of smoking on these newborn parameters.

Placenta is an important organ for nutrients and oxygen exchanges between mother and fetus. Determinants of placenta growth however are still largely unknown. It is likely that smoking induces negative effects on placental structure with alterations in vascularization that could be responsible for the decrease of BW and for the slight decrease of PW. It has been reported that smoking interferes with the proliferation of placental cells and with the rate of cell death [1, 15].

It has been suggested that the decreased function of placenta in relation to fetal request may induce a slight compensatory increase of PW to provide nutritional support and efficient oxygen exchange for the fetus [14].

Our study suggests that environmental and probably also genetic differences between populations could modulate the effects of smoking on intrauterine development.

In Penne the population is homogeneous: these people are descendant of an old italic population called "Vestini" while in Rome the population is composed by immigrants from all regions of Italy. Because of the Valund effect the heterogeneity of Rome population could result in an increase of homozygous genotypes in Rome as compared to Penne. Indeed we have tested this effect in ABO, ACP_1 and PGM_1 genetic polymorphisms and found an increase of homozygous genotypes in Rome as compared to Penne (see Table 1). Homozygosity could increase the susceptibility to damaging effects of toxic substances.

Environmental differences between Penne and Rome, however, may have a more important role. In the rural area of Penne environmental pollution is practically absent while in the urban area of Rome the pollution is high. Environmental pollution may have an additive effect with cigarette smoking concerning the unfavorable effect on intrauterine development. In Penne the winters are very cold while in Rome are very mild. Low environmental temperature may contribute to increase the metabolic output enhancing the defense against toxic substances of cigarette smoking.

Alimentary factors may also have an important role. Natural foods without pesticides are more available in a rural than in a metropolitan environment and these differences may contribute to lower the effect of smoking on intrauterine growth observed in the population of Penne.

The effect of maternal age could be related to a cumulative effect of smoking on reproductive performance resulting in a more evident effect of cigarette smoking in the offspring of older women.

References

[1] Jauniaux, E. & Burton, G. J. (2007). Morphological and biological effects of maternal exposure to tobacco smoke on the feto-placental unit. *Early Hum Dev*, *83*,699-706.

[2] Cliver, S. P., Goldenberg, R. L., Cutter, G. R., et al. (1995). The effect of cigarette smoking on neonatal anthropometric measurements. *Obstet Gynecol*, *85*,625-30.

[3] Hrubá, D. & Kachlík, P. (2000). Influence of maternal active and passive smoking during pregnancy on birthweight in newborns. *Cent Eur J Public Health*, *8*, 249-52.

[4] Ohmi, H., Hirooka, K. & Mochizuki, Y. (2002). Fetal growth and the timing of exposure to maternal smoking. *Pediatr Int*, *44*, 55-9.

[5] Steyn, K., de Wet, T., Saloojee, Y., et al. (2006). The influence of maternal cigarette smoking, snuff use and passive smoking on pregnancy outcomes: the Birth To Ten Study. *Paediatr Perinat Epidemiol*, *20*, 90-9.

[6] Walfisch, A., Nikolovski, S., Talevska, B. & Hallak, M. (2013). Fetal growth *Arch Gynecol Obstet.*, *287*, 1131-6.

[7] McNamara, H., Hutcheon, J. A., Platt, R. W., Benjamin, A. & Kramer, M. S. (2014). Risk factors for high and low placental weight. *Paediatr Perinat Epidemiol.*, 28,97-105.

[8] Williams, L. A., Evans, S. F. & Newnham, J. P. (1997). Prospective cohort study of factors influencing the relative weights of the placenta and the newborn infant. *BMJ*, *314*, 1864-8.

[9] Belkacemi, L., Nelson, D. M., Desai, M., et al. (2010). Maternal undernutrition influences placental-fetal development. *Biol Reprod*, *83*, 325-31.

[10] Burton, G. J., Jauniaux, E., Charnock-Jones, D. S. (2010). The influence of the intrauterine environment on human placental development. *Int J Dev Biol*, *54*, 303-12.

[11] Winder, N. R., Krishnaveni, G. V., Veena, S. R. et al. (2011). Mother's lifetime nutrition and the size, shape and efficiency of the placenta. *Placenta*, *32*, 806-10.

[12] Salafia, C. M., Zhang, J., Charles, A. K., et al. (2008). Placental characteristics and birthweight. Paediatr Perinat Epidemiol, 22,229-39.

[13] Rizzo, G., Capponi, A., Pietrolucci, M. E., et al. (2009). Effects of maternal cigarette smoking on placental volume and vascularization

measured by 3-dimensional power Doppler ultrasonography at 11+0 to 13+6 weeks of gestation. *Am J Obstet Gynecol*, *200*, 415e1-5.

[14] Wang, N., Tikellis, G., Sun, C., et al. (2014). The effect of maternal prenatal smoking and alcohol consumption on the placenta-to-birth weight ratio. *Placenta*, *35*, 437-41.

[15] Genbacev, O., McMaster, M. T., Lazic, J., et al. (2000). Concordant in situ and in vitro data show that maternal cigarette smoking negatively regulates placental cytotrophoblast passage through the cell cycle. *Reprod Toxicol*, *14*, 495-506.

In: Macrosomia and Birth Weight
Editor: Larry P. Harris

ISBN: 978-1-63483-124-6

Chapter V

Bibliography

Golden hours: care of the very low birth weight infant LCCN: 2014940198 Type of material: Book Personal name: Bissinger, Robin Louise. Main title: Golden hours: care of the very low birth weight infant / [edited by] Robin L. Bissinger, Phd, APRN, NNP-BC, FAAN, Associate Dean of Academics, Neonatal Nurse Practitioner, College of Nursing, Medical University of South Carolina, Carleston, South Carolina, David J. Annibale, MD, Chief, Division of Neonatology, Program Director, Fellowship in Neonatal-Perinatal Medicine, Children's Hospital, Division of Neonatology, Medical University of South Carolina, Carleston, South Carolina. Edition: First edition. Published/Created: Chicago: The National Certification Corporation, 2014. Description: xv, 400 pages: illustrations (chiefly color); 19 cm. ISBN: 9780989019811 0989019810 LC classification: RJ250 .B57 2014 Portion of title: Care of the very low birth weight infant Related names: Annibale, David J. Contents: Fetal assessment / Carol Burke and Catherine Theorell - Maternal risk factors / Catherine Theorell - Neonatal assessment / Terri A. Cavaliere - Transition at birth and umbilical cord blood gas analysis / Gautham K. Suresh - Basic management of the airway / Catherine Theorell - Cardiac support / Catherine Theorell - Thermoregulation / Robin L. Bissinger - Respiratory diseases / Frances R. Koch - Pulmonary emergencies / Cheryl A. Carlson

- Cardiovascular stability and shock / Lyn Vargo - Cardiac emergencies / Julie R. Ross - Fluids, electrolytes, and nutrition / Jan Sherman - Hypoglycemia / Jan Sherman - Neonatal sepsis / Jan Sherman - Intraventricular hemorrhage / Bresney Crowell and David J. Annibale - Hematologic emergencies / James R. Kiger - Surgical emergencies: abdominal wall defects / Robin L. Bissinger and Ellen Tappero - Congenital anomalies / Ellen Tappero - Developmentally supportive and family-centered care / Jacqueline M. McGrath, Ana Francisca Diallo, Rebecca J. Paquette, and Haifa (Abou) Samra - Ethical dilemmas / Margaret Conway-Orgel - Teamwork and communication / Margaret Conway-Orgel - Neonatal transport / Fran Byrd - Procedural review / Cheryl A. Carlson - Appendix A. Resource toolbox. I. Fetal assessment: Fetal lung maturity; Reference values for umbilical cord blood gas values; Umbilical sampling - II. Respiratory system: Targeted saturation goal in the first 10 min of life; Apgar scoring at birth; Initial positive-pressure ventilation (PPV); Intubation guidelines - III. Thermoregulation: Recommended axillary temperatures in infants [less than or equal to sign] 1,500 grams; Recommended stabilization room temperatures based on post-menstrual age and birth weight; Example of humidity guidelines - IV. Cardiovascular system: Treatment of hypotension; Recommended volume expanders in the delivery room - V. Fluids and electrolytes: Suggested response to blood glucose [less than or equal to sign] 45 mg/dL or symptomatic (example of a protocol) - VI. Neurological system: Grading of intraventricular hemorrhage (IVH) - VIII. Procedures: Umbilical line measurements and placement - VIII. Web resources - Appendix B. Glossary of acronyms. Subjects: Neonatal intensive care. Premature infants. Notes: Includes bibliographical references and index. Dewey class no.: 618.92/01

Low-birthweight baby: born too soon or too small LCCN: 2014044139 Type of material: Book Meeting name: Nestlé Nutrition Workshop (81st: 2014: Magaliesburg, South Africa), author. Main title: Low-birthweight baby: born too soon or too small / editors, Nicholas D. Embleton, Joanne Katz,

Ekhard E. Ziegler. Published/Produced: Basel, Switzerland; New York: Karger; Vevey, Switzerland: Nestlé Nutrition Institute, [2015] Projected pub date: 1502 Description: p.; cm. ISBN: 9783318027686 (hard cover: alk. paper) LC classification: RJ281 Related names: Embleton, Nicholas D., editor. Katz, Joanne, editor. Ziegler, Ekhard E., editor. Subjects: Infant, Low Birth Weight--Congresses. Infant Nutritional Physiological Phenomena--Congresses. Infant, Premature--Congresses. Notes: Includes bibliographical references and index. Series: Nestlé Nutrition Institute workshop series, 1664-2147; vol. 81 Nestlé Nutrition Institute workshop series; v. 81. 1664-2147 Dewey class no.: 618.92/011

Maternal and child nutrition: the first 1,000 days LCCN: 2013015233 Type of material: Book Meeting name: Nestlé Nutrition Workshop (74th: 2012: Velha Goa, India) Main title: Maternal and child nutrition: the first 1,000 days / editors, Jatinder Bhatia, Zulfiqar A. Bhutta, Satish C. Kalhan. Published/Created: Basel: Karger; Vevey, Switzerland: Nestlé Nutrition Institute, c2013. Description: xvii, 237 p.: ill.; 25 cm. ISBN: 9783318023879 (hbk.: acid-free paper) LC classification: RJ250.3 .N47 2012 Related names: Bhatia, Jatinder, 1952- Bhutta, Zulfiqar Ahmed, 1955- Kalhan, Satish C. Nestlé Nutrition Institute. Subjects: Infant Nutrition Disorders--prevention & control. Infant, Low Birth Weight--growth & development. Infant Nutritional Physiological Phenomena. Maternal Nutritional Physiological Phenomena. Nutritional Requirements. Notes: Includes bibliographical references and index. Series: Nestlé Nutrition Institute workshop series, 1664-2147; vol. 74 Nestlé Nutrition Institute workshop series; v. 74. 1664-2147 Dewey class no.: 618.92/011

Nutritional care of preterm infants: scientific basis and practical guidelines LCCN: 2014007369 Type of material: Book Main title: Nutritional care of preterm infants: scientific basis and practical guidelines / volume editors, Berthold Koletzko, M unich, Brenda Poindexter, Indianapolis, Ind., Ricardo Uauy, Santiago de Chile. Published/Produced: Basel: Karger, [2014] ©2014 Description: xii, 314 pages:

illustrations (some color); 26 cm. ISBN: 9783318026405 (hard cover: alk. paper) 3318026409 (hard cover: alk. paper) LC classification: RJ216 .N8598 2014 Related names: Koletzko, B. (Berthold), editor. Poindexter, Brenda, editor. Uauy, Ricardo, editor. Contents: Historical perspective / R.C. Tsang - Defining the nutritional needs of preterm infants / R. Uauy, B. Koletzko - Nutrition, growth and clinical outcomes / R.A. Ehrenkranz - Assessing the evidence from neonatal nutrition research / H. Szajewska, B. Koletzko, F. Mimouni, R. Uauy - Amino acids and proteins / J.B. van Goudoever, H. Vlaardingerbroek, C.H. van den Akker, F. de Groof, S.R.D. van der Schoor - Energy requirements, protein-energy metabolism and balance, and carbohydrates in preterm infants / W.W. Hay Jr., L.D. Brown, S.C. Denne - Lipids / A. Lapillonne - Water, sodium, potassium and chloride / C. Fusch, F. Jochum - Nutritional care of premature infants: microminerals / M. Domellf - Calcium, phosphorus, magnesium and vitamin d requirements of the preterm infant / F.B. Mimouni, D. Mandel, R. Lubetzky, T. Senterre - Vitamins - conventional uses and new insights / A. Leaf, Z. Lansdowne - The developing intestinal microbiome: probiotics and prebiotics / J. Neu - Practice of parenteral nutrition in vlbw and elbw infants / N.D. Embleton, K. Simmer - Preterm nutrition and the brain / S.E. Ramel, M.K. Georgieff - Practice of enteral nutrition in very low birth weight and extremely low birth weight infants / T. Senterre - Human milk and human milk fortifiers / E.E. Ziegler - Approaches to growth faltering / B.B. Poindexter - Preterm nutrition and the lung / F. Moya - Necrotizing enterocolitis / J. Neu - Feeding after discharge / A. Lapillonne - Meeting the challenge of providing neonatal nutritional care to very or extremely low birth weight infants in low-resource settings / T. Murguia-Peniche, G.F. Kirsten - Recommended nutrient intake levels for stable, fully enterally fed very low birth weight infants / B. Koletzko, B. Poindexter, R. Uauy. Subjects: Infant, Premature. Infant Care. Infant Nutritional Physiological Phenomena. Notes: Includes bibliographical references and index. Series: World review of nutrition and dietetics, 0084-2230; vol. 110 World review of nutrition and dietetics; v. 110.

0084-2230 Dewey class no.: 618.92/01

Perinatal programming: the state of the art LCCN: 2011022261 Type of material: Book Main title: Perinatal programming: the state of the art / edited by Andreas Plagemann. Published/Created: Berlin; Boston: De Gruyter, c2012. Description: xv, 293 p.: ill. (some col.); 25 cm. ISBN: 9783110249446 (alk. paper) 9783110249453 (e-ISBN) LC classification: RG600 .P47 2012 Related names: Plagemann, Andreas. Contents: The past and future of perinatal medicine - Experimental models of low birth weight--insight into the developmental programming of metabolic health, aging, and immune function - Cardiovascular consequences of IUGR: experimental aspects - Fetal programming of endocrine function in IUGR offspring depends on the cause of low birth weight: evidence from animal models and the human FIPS-study - Intrauterine corticosteroids for lung maturation: observations of HPA axis function and cardiac autonomic balance in the neonate - Feast or famine: in the fast lane to puberty - Early life origins of diabetes and obesity: general aspects and the thin-fat baby paradigm - The outcome in offspring of obese mothers - Short and long term effects of gestational obesity: clinical observations - Emerging role of neuroendocrine programming in obesity - Genetic influences on the long-term effects of the perinatal environment on energy homeostasis and offspring obesity - Perinatal programming in offspring of diabetic mothers: clinical data - Experimental observations on perinatal programming in offspring of diabetic mothers - Prenatal infections and long-term mental outcome: modeling schizophrenia-related dysfunctions using the prenatal Poly I: C model in mice - Prenatal programming of cognition and emotion in humans: from birth to age 20 - Perinatal programming of allergy - Perinatal origin of testicular germ cell cancer: possible involvement of developmental re-programming - Epigenetic adaptation during early life - Toward a unifying concept on perinatal programming: vegetative imprinting by environment-dependent biocybernetogenesis. Subjects: Perinatology. Prenatal Exposure Delayed Effects. Perinatology--trends. Notes:

Includes bibliographical references and indexes. Dewey class no.: 618.3/2

Textbook of children's environmental health LCCN: 2013026015 Type of material: Book Main title: Textbook of children's environmental health / [edited by] Philip J. Landrigan and Ruth A. Etzel. Published/Produced: Oxford; New York, NY: Oxford University Press, [2014] Description: xviii, 588 p.: illustrations; 27 cm. ISBN: 9780199929573 (alk. paper) LC classification: RJ102 .T49 2014 Related names: Landrigan, Philip J., editor of compilation. Etzel, Ruth Ann, editor of compilation. Contents: Children's environmental health: a new branch of pediatrics / Philip J. Landrigan and Ruth A. Etzel - Children's exquisite vulnerability to environmental exposures / Ruth A. Etzel and Philip J. Landrigan - The chemical environment and children's health / Philip J. Landrigan and Ruth A. Etzel - Intrauterine nutrition and children's health / Robert H. Lane, Lisa Joss-Moore, Ryann Bierer, Laurie J. Moyer-Mileur - Social and behavioral influences on child health and development / Rosalind J. Wright - Epidemiology a tool for studying environmental influences on children's health / Dean Baker - Exposure science to protect children's health / Paul J. Lioy and Clifford P. Weisel - Geographic information systems (GIS) in children's environmental health / Panos G. Georgopoulos and Paul J. Lioy - Developmental toxicology and children's environmental health / Edward D. Levin - Genetics, epigenetics, and children's environmental health / Robert O. Wright - Economics and children's environmental health / Philip J. Landrigan - The global dimension of children's environmental health / Ruth A. Etzel - The intrauterine environment and early infancy / Ami Zota, Dylan Atchley, Tracey Woodruff - The home environment / Johnna S. Murphy and Megan Sandel - The school/child care environment / Mana Mann and Maida Galvez - The shape of the built environment shapes children's health / Richard J. Jackson and Ashley Kissinger - The play environment / James Roberts, James T. McElligott, Kristina Kay Gustafson - The benefits of the green environment / William Crain and Ellen F. Crain - The farm environment / James A. Merchant and Diane S. Rohlman

- Workplace safety for young workers / Carol W. Runyan, Michael D. Schulman, and Lawrence E. Scholl - The changing global environment and children's health / Perry E. Sheffield and Kristie L. Ebi - Outdoor air pollution / Douglas W. Dockery - Indoor air pollution / Archana Patel - Tobacco smoke: active and passive / Jonathan M. Samet - Water pollution / Tim Ford and Steve Hamner - Sanitation and hygiene / Ruth A. Etzel - Hazardous waste and toxic hotspots / Richard Fuller - Lead / Bruce Lanphear - Mercury / Philippe Grandjean - Arsenic / Fen Wu, Faruque Parvez, Joseph H. Graziano, and Yu Chen - Other metals / Roberto Lucchini and Chiara Benedetti - Pesticides / Catherine J. Karr and Virginia A. Rauh - PCBs, dioxins, furans, DDT, polybrominated compounds, polyfluorinated compounds, and other halogenated hydrocarbons / Philip J. Landrigan - Volatile organic chemicals / Dana Boyd Barr, P. Barry Ryan, and Brian Buckley - Endocrine disruptors / Annemarie Stroustrup and Shanna H. Swan - Chemical obesogens and obesity / Michele La Merrill, Kyla Taylor, Kristina A. Thayer, and Linda S. Birnbaum - Environmental carcinogens and childhood cancer / Irena Buka and Alvaro Osornio - Mold / Dorr G. Dearborn - Physical hazards / Sophie J. Balk - Ionizing radiation / David Hoel - Electromagnetic fields / Kurt Straiff, Robert Baan, Neela Guha - Prematurity, low birth weight, and the environment / Shiv Kapoor and Cynthia F. Bearer - Asthma, allergy, and the environment / Peter D. Sly - Neurodevelopmental disorders and the environment / David C. Bellinger - Birth defects and the environment / Christina Chambers - Obesity, diabetes, cardiovascular disease, and the environment / Nikki Mihalopoulos - Liver disease in children and the environment / Frederick J. Suchy - Kidney disease in children and the environment / Virginia M. Weaver - Injuries, trauma, and the environment / Catherine J. Vladutiu and Renee M. Johnson - Acute pediatric poisoning / Jennifer Lowry - The environmental history & examination: the key to diagnosis of environmental diseases / Jerome A. Paulson and Lauren Gordon - Clinical practice of environmental pediatrics around the world / Amalia Laborde - Public policy on children's environmental health in the United States / Lynn Goldman and Philip J. Landrigan - Public policy on children's environmental health in the Europe / Genon K. Jensen and Diana G. Smith - Public policy on childrens environmental health in Asia / Eunhee Ha - Global treaties and children's environmental health / Roberto Bertollini - The impact of poverty, disparity, and injustice on children's environmental health / Luz Claudio - War, terrorism, and children's health / Barry S. Levy and Victor W. Sidel - Natural disasters, environmental emergencies and children's health / Henry Falk - New frontiers in children's environmental health / Philip J. Landrigan, and Ruth A. Etzel. Subjects: Child--United States. Environmental Health--United States. Environmental Exposure--adverse effects--United States. Environmental Pollutants--adverse effects--United States. Notes: Includes bibliographical references and index. Dewey class no.: 362.19892

The new public health LCCN: 2014427175 Type of material: Book Personal name: Tulchinsky, Theodore H., author. Main title: The new public health / Theodore H. Tulchinsky, MD, MPH, Braun School of Public Health, Hebrew University-Hadassah, Ein Karem, Jerusalem, Israel and Elena A. Varavikova, MD, MPH, PhD, Research Institute for Public Health Organization and Information (CNIIOIZ), Moscow, Russian Federation with Joan D. Bickford, MSN, Former Chief Public Health Nurse, Province of Manitoba, Canada; foreword by Jonathan Fielding, MD, MPH, University of Los Angeles (UCLA), California. Edition: Third edition. Published/Produced: Amsterdam; Boston: Elsevier/AP, [2014] ©2014 Description: xxv, 884 pages: illustrations; 28 cm ISBN: 9780124157668 (hbk) 0124157661 (hbk) LC classification: RA425 .T77 2014 Related names: Varavikova, Elena, author. Bickford, Joan D., author. Summary: The book provides a unified approach to public health appropriate for all masters' level students and practitioners-specifically for courses in MPH programs, community health and preventive medicine programs, community health education programs, community health nursing programs. Contents: Machine generated contents note: 1.A History of Public

Health - Introduction - Prehistoric Societies - The Ancient World - The Early Medieval Period (Fifth to Tenth Centuries CE) - The Late Medieval Period (Eleventh to Fifteenth Centuries) - The Renaissance (1400--1600s) - Enlightenment, Science, and Revolution (1600s--1800s) - Eighteenth-Century Reforms - Applied Epidemiology - Jenner and Vaccination - Foundations of Health Statistics and Epidemiology - Social Reform and the Sanitary Movement (1830--1875) - Social Security - Snow on Cholera - The Germ and Miasma Theories - Hospital Reform - The Bacteriological Revolution - Pasteur, Cohn, Koch, and Lister - The Basis of Genetics - Vectorborne Disease - Microbiology and Immunology - Poliomyelitis - Advances in Prevention and Treatment of Infectious Diseases - Infections and Chronic Diseases - Maternal and Child Health - Nutrition in Public Health - Military Medicine - Globalization of Health - Contents note continued: Epidemiological Transition - Achievements of Public Health in the Twentieth Century - Creating and Managing Health Systems - Challenges in the Twenty-First Century - Summary - Historical Markers - Note - Bibliography - 2.Expanding the Concept of Public Health - Introduction - Concepts of Public Health - Evolution of Public Health - Health and Disease - The Host-Agent--Environment Paradigm - The Expanded Host-Agent-Environment Paradigm - The Natural History of Disease - Society and Health - Health Insurance Systems - Health Promotion - Social Determinants of Health - Modes of Prevention - Health Promotion - Health Protection - Primary Prevention - Secondary Prevention - Tertiary Prevention - Demographic and Epidemiological Transition - Interdependence of Health Services - Defining Public Health - Social Medicine and Community Health - Social Hygiene, Eugenics, and Corruption of Public Health Concepts - Medical Ecology - Contents note continued: Community-Oriented Primary Care - The World Health Organization's Definition of Health - Alma-Ata: Health for All - Selective Primary Care - The Risk Approach - The Case for Action - Political Economy and Health - Social, Behavioral, and Political Sciences - Health and Development - Health Systems: The Case for Reform -

Advocacy and Consumerism - Professional Advocacy and Resistance - Consumerism - The Health Field Concept - The Value of Medical Care in Public Health - Health Targets - US Health Targets - European Health Targets - UK Health Targets - Individual and Community Participation in Health - Founding of Health Promotion: The Ottawa Charter of 1986 - State and Community Models of Health Promotion - Healthy Cities/Towns/Municipalities - Human Ecology and Health Promotion - Defining Public Health Standards - Integrative Approaches to Public Health - Achievements of Public Health - The Future of Public Health - Contents note continued: The New Public Health - Summary - Note - Bibliography - 3.Measuring, Monitoring, and Evaluating the Health of a Population - Introduction - Demography - Fertility - Population Pyramid - Life Expectancy - Epidemiology - Social Epidemiology - Epidemiology in Building Health Policy - Definitions and Methods of Epidemiology - Rates and Ratios - Measures of Disease Occurrence or Morbidity - Prevalence Rates - Measures of Mortality - Social Classification - Sentinel Events - The Burden of Disease - Years of Potential Life Lost - Qualitative Measures of Morbidity and Mortality - Measurement - Research and Survey Methods - Variables - The Null Hypothesis - Confounders - Sampling - Random Sampling - Normal Distribution - Standardization of Rates - Direct Method of Standardization - Indirect Method of Standardization - Potential Errors in Measurement - Reliability - Validity - Screening for Disease - Epidemiological Studies - Contents note continued: Observational Studies - Experimental Epidemiology - Establishing Causal Relationships - Notification of Diseases - Special Registries and Reporting Systems - Disease Classification - Hospital Discharge Information - Health Information Systems (Informatics) - WHO European Region Health for All Database - Surveillance, Reporting, and Publication - Assessing the Health of the Individual - Assessment of Population Health - Defining the Population - Health Care Financing and Organization - Health Care Resources - Utilization of Services - Health Care

Outcomes - Quality of Care - Self-Assessment of Health - Costs and Benefits - Effects of Intervention - Qualitative and Quantitative Research Methods - From Health Information to Knowledge to Policy - Summary - Note - Bibliography - 4.Communicable Diseases - Introduction - Public Health and the Control of Communicable Disease - The Nature of Communicable Disease - Contents note continued: Host-Agent-Environment Triad - Classifications of Communicable Diseases - Modes of Transmission of Disease - Immunity - Surveillance - Healthcare-Associated Infections - Endemic and Epidemic Disease - Epidemic Investigation - Control of Communicable Diseases - Treatment - Methods of Prevention - Vaccine-Preventable Diseases - Immunization Coverage - Vaccine Regulation, Schedules, and Programs - Essentials of an Immunization Program - Regulation of Vaccines - Vaccine Development - Connections Between Infectious and Chronic Diseases - Control and Eradication of Infectious Diseases - Success in Eradicating Smallpox - Eradication of Poliomyelitis - Future Candidates for Disease - Eradication - Criteria for Eradicable Diseases - Directly Observed Therapy Short Course (DOTS) - Vectorborne Diseases - Malaria - Rickettsial Infections - Arboviruses (Arthropod-Borne Viral Diseases) - Lyme Disease - Neglected Tropical Diseases - Contents note continued: Echinococcosis - Tapeworm - Onchocerciasis - Dracunculiasis - Schistosomiasis - Leishmaniasis - Trypanosomiasis - Other Parasitic Diseases - Legionnaire's Disease - Leprosy - Sexually Transmitted Infections - Syphilis - Gonorrhea - Chancroid - Herpes Simplex - Chlamydia - Trachoma - Trichomoniasis - Human Papillomavirus - Control of Sexually Transmitted Infections - HIV/AIDS - Diarrheal Diseases - Salmonella - Shigella - Escherichia coli - Cholera - Viral Gastroenteritis - Parasitic Gastroenteritis - A Program Approach to Diarrheal Disease Control - Acute Respiratory Infections - Inequalities in Control of Communicable Diseases - Communicable Disease Control in the New Public Health - Summary - Note - Bibliography - 5.Non-Communicable Diseases and Conditions - Introduction - The

Rise and Spread of Chronic Disease - Environment and Lifestyle - Global Burden of Mortality - Contents note continued: Risk Factors, Health Promotion, and Prevention of Non-Communicable Diseases - Tobacco - Alcohol and Other Drugs - Physical Activity - Hypertension - Diet and Obesity - Mental Illness - Genetic, Infectious, and Non-Communicable Diseases - The Social and Economic Burden of Non-Communicable Diseases - Health Promotion and Disease Prevention - Hypertension and Cardiovascular Diseases - Diabetes Mellitus - Prevention of Diabetes and Its Complications - Cancer - Prevention of Carton - Trauma, Violence, and Injury - Motor Vehicle Accidents - Domestic and Sexual Violence - Suicide - Poisoning - Homicide - Prevention of Violence - Chronic Lung Disease - Asthma - Chronic Obstructive Pulmonary Disease - Restrictive Lung Diseases - Occupational Lung Diseases - End-Stage Renal Disease - Disabling Conditions - Arthritis and Musculoskeletal Disorders - Osteoporosis - Degenerative Osteoarthritis - Rheumatoid Arthritis and Gout - Contents note continued: Low Back and Neck Pain Syndromes - Neurological Disorders - Alzheimer's Disease - Parkinson's Disease - Multiple Sclerosis - Epilepsy or Seizures - Brain and Spinal Cord Injury - Visual Disorders - Hearing Disorders - Non-Communicable Diseases and the New Public Health - Integrated Non-Communicable Disease Prevention and Control - Summary - Note - Bibliography - Recommended Reading - Global Burden of Non-Communicable - Diseases - Social Determinants, Environment, and Economics of Non-Communicable Diseases - Risk Factors, Health Promotion, and Prevention of Non-Communicable Diseases - Smoking - Diet, Physical Activity, and Obesity - Infectious Diseases and Non-Communicable Diseases - Hypertension and Cardiovascular Diseases - Metabolic Syndrome, Diabetes Mellitus, and End-Stage Renal Disease - Cancer - Trauma, Violence, Injury, and Suicide - Chronic Lung Disease - Disabling Conditions - 6.Family Health - Introduction - Contents note continued: The Family Unit - Preventive Health through Life Stages - The Family Physician Cannot do All This Alone -

Maternal Health - Fertility - Public Health Challenges of Fertility - Family Planning - Maternal Mortality and Morbidity - Pregnancy Care - High-Risk Pregnancy - Labor and Delivery - Safe Motherhood Initiatives - Care of the Newborn - Low Birth Weight/Preterm Birth - Postdelivery Care (Puerperium) - Genetic and Birth Disorders - Rhesus Hemolytic Disease of the Newborn - Neural Tube Defects - Cerebral Palsy - Low Birth Weight and Developmental Disability - Down Syndrome - Cystic Fibrosis - Sickle-Cell Disease - Thalassemia - Phenylketonuria - Congenital Hypothyroidism - Congenital Syphilis - Fetal Alcohol Syndrome - Tay--Sachs Disease - Glucose-6-Phosphate Dehydrogenase Deficiency - Familial Mediterranean Fever - Infant and Child Health - Fetal and Infant Mortality - Infancy Care and Feeding - Contents note continued: Anticipatory Counseling - Documentation, Records, and Monitoring - Preschool Children (Age 1--5 Years) - School and Adolescent Health - Smoking - Alcohol Abuse - Drug Abuse - Sexual Risk Behavior - Dietary Risk Behavior - Physical Activity - Violence and Gang Behavior - Adult Health - Women's Health - Men's Health - Health of Older Adults - Health Maintenance for Older Adults - Summary - Note - Bibliography - 7.Special Community Health Needs - Introduction - Mental Health - Historical Changes in Methods of Treatment - Mental Health Epidemiology - Mental Disorder Syndromes - Controversies in Mental Health Policies - Community-Oriented Mental Health - Prevention and Health Promotion - Intellectual Disability - Oral Health - Fluoridation - Periodontal Disease - Dental Care - Oral Cancer - Physical Disability and Rehabilitation - Special Croup Health Needs - Cay and Lesbian Health - Native Peoples' Health - Contents note continued: Prisoners' Health - Migrant Population Health - Homeless Population Health - Refugee Health - Military Medicine - Health in Disasters - Summary - Note - Bibliography - Mental Health - Oral Health - Disability and Rehabilitation - Cay and Lesbian Health - Native Peoples' Health - Prisoners' Health - Migrant and Refugee Health - Military Medicine - Disasters and Health - 8.Nutrition and Food Safety - Introduction - Development of Nutrition in Public Health - Nutrition in a

Global Context - Nutrition and Infection - Functions of Food - Human Nutritional Requirements - Carbohydrates - Proteins - Fats and Oils - Vitamins - Minerals and Trace Elements - Growth - Measuring Body Mass - Recommended Dietary Intakes - Disorders of Undernutrition - Underweight: Protein---Energy Malnutrition - Failure to Thrive - Marasmus - Kwashiorkor - Micronutrient Deficiencies - Osteoporosis - Eating Disorders - Diseases of Overnutrition - Contents note continued: Overweight/Obesity - Diabetes Mellitus - Cardiovascular Diseases - Cancer - Nutrition in Pregnancy and Lactation - Promoting Healthy Diets and Lifestyles - Dietary Guidelines - Vitamin and Mineral Enrichment of Basic Foods - Controversy in Food Enrichment - Genetically Modified Foods - Food and Nutrition Policy - Evolution of a Federal Role - Nutrition Issues in Development Policies - Role of the Private Sector and Non-Governmental Organizations - Role of Health Providers - Nutrition Monitoring and Evaluation - Standard Reference Populations - Measuring Deviation from the Reference Population - Global Nutrition Targets for 2025 - Food Quality and Safety - Nutrition and the New Public Health - Summary - Note - Bibliography - Recommended Reading - Foodborne Illness, Nutrition, and Infectious Disease - Monitoring Growth and Body Mass - Nutrient Requirements, Recommended Dietary Intakes, and Dietary Guidelines - Contents note continued: Micronutrient Deficiency Conditions - Vitamin D and Bone Health - Nutrition, Obesity, and Chronic Disease - Maternal/Child Nutrition and Survival - Food Fortification - Food and Nutrition Policy, and Food Security - Nutrition Monitoring and Evaluation - 9.Environmental and Occupational Health - Environmental Health - Introduction - Global Environmental Issues - Geographic and Environmental Epidemiology - Environmental Targets - Environment and Infectious Diseases - Global Climate Change - Environmental Impact on Health Burden of Disease - Community Water Supplies - Waterborne Diseases - Waterborne Disease Surveillance and Prevalence, USA - Water as a Global Resource - Sewage Collection and Treatment - Solid Waste - Toxins - Toxic Effects on

Fertility - Toxic Effects of Lead in the Environment - Agricultural and Environmental Hazards - Air Pollution - The External Environment - Methyl Tertiary Butyl Ether - Indoor Pollution - Contents note continued: Effects of Indoor Air Pollution - Radon Gas - Outdoor--Indoor Pollutants - Biological Pollutants - Built Environment and Health - Hazardous or Toxic Wastes - Minimata Disease - Toxic Waste Management - Radiation - Ionizing Radiation - Non-Ionizing Radiation - Environmental Impact - Emergency Events Involving Hazardous Substances - Human-Caused Disasters - War, Terrorism, and Genocide - Preventing and Managing Environmental Emergencies - Environmental Health Organization - Occupational Health - Introduction - Development of Occupational Health - The Health of Workers - The Burden of Occupational Morbidity and Mortality - Occupational Health Priorities in the USA - International Issues in Occupational Health - National and Management Responsibilities - Standards and Monitoring - Occupational Health Targets - Occupational Injury - Toxicity at the Workplace and in the Environment - Lead - Asbestos - Silica - Contents note continued: Cotton Dust (Byssinosis) - Vinyl Chloride - Agent Orange - Workplace Violence - Occupational Health in Clinical Practice - Inspecting the Place of Work - Risk Assessment - Preventing Disasters in the Workplace - Occupation and The New Public Health - Summary - Note - Bibliography - Environmental Health - Occupational Health - 10.Organization of Public Health Systems - Introduction - Government and Health of the Nation - Federal and Unitary States - Checks and Balances in Health Authority - Government and the Individual - Functions of Public Health - Regulatory Functions of Public Health Agencies - Investigative Functions of Public Health - Prevention of Injuries - Methods of Providing or Assuring Services: Direct or Indirect? - Non-Governmental Roles in Health - Disasters and Public Health Preparedness - Medical Practice and Public Health - Incentives and Regulation - Promotion of Research and Teaching - Contents note continued: Accreditation and Quality Regulation - National Government Public Health

Services - State Government Public Health Services - Local Health Authorities - Accreditation of Public Health Departments - Monitoring Health Status - National Health Targets - Universal Health Coverage and the New Public Health - Hospitals in the New Public Health - Hospital Classification - Supply of Hospital Beds - The Changing Role of the Hospital - Innovations in Health Care Delivery - The Uninsured as a Public Health Challenge - US Patient Protection and Affordable Care Act (Obamacare) - Summary - Note - Bibliography - Agencies and Organizations - Recommended Reading - 11.Measuring Costs: The Economics of Health - Introduction - Economic Issues of Health Systems - Investing in Health - Basic Concepts in Health Economics - Supply, Need, Demand, and Utilization of Health Services - Normative Needs - Felt Need - Expressed Need - Comparative Need - Contents note continued: Demand - Supply - Grossman's Demand Model - Competition in Health Care - Elasticities of Demand - Measuring Costs - Economic Measures of Health Status - Cost--Benefit Analysis - Cost-Effectiveness Analysis - Basic Assessment Scheme for Intervention Costs and Consequences - The Value of Human Life - Health Financing: The Macroeconomic Level - Costs of Illness - Costs and Variations in Medical Practice - Cost Containment - Medical and Hospital Care: Microeconomics - Payment for Doctors' Services - Payment for Comprehensive Care - Health Maintenance and Managed Care Organizations - District Health Systems - Paying for Hospital Care - Capital Costs - Hospital Supply, Utilization, and Costs - Modified Market Forces - Economics of Prevention - Game Theory, Economics, and Health Policy - Economics and the New Public Health - Summary - Note - Bibliography - 12.Planning and Managing Health Systems - Introduction - Contents note continued: Health Policy and Planning as Context - The Elements of Organizations - Scientific Management - Bureaucratic Pyramidal Organizations - Organizations as Energy Systems - Cybernetics and Management - Target-Oriented Management - Operations Research - Management by Objectives - Human Relations Management - The Hawthorne Effect - Maslow's Hierarchy of Needs -

Theory X--Theory Y - Network Organization - Total Quality Management - Changing Human Behavior - Empowerment - Strategic Management of Health Systems - Health System Organization Models - Functional Model - Corporate Model - Matrix Model - Skills for Management - The Chief Executive Officer of Health Organizations - Community Participation - Integration: Lateral and Vertical - Norms and Performance Indicators - Health Promotion and Advocacy - Philanthropy and Volunteerism - New Organizational Models - New Projects and their Evaluation - Contents note continued: Competencies in Health Policy and Management - Systems Approach and National Planning - Summary - Note - Bibliography - Electronic Resources - Recommended Reading - 13.National Health Systems - Introduction - Health Systems in the Industrialized Countries - Evolution of Health Systems - Social Insurance - National Health Service - National Health Insurance - The United States - Federal Health Initiatives - Medicare and Medicaid - The Changing Health Care Environment - Health Information - Health Targets - Social Inequalities - The Dilemma of the Uninsured - Summary - Canada - Reform Pressures and Initiatives - Provincial Health Reforms - Health Status - Summary - The United Kingdom - The National Health Service - Reforms in the 1970s and 1980s - Reforms Since 1990 - Social and Regional Inequalities - Health Promotion - Health Reforms - Primary Care Trusts - Summary - The Nordic Countries - Sweden - Denmark - Contents note continued: Norway - Finland - Western Europe - Germany - The Netherlands - Russia - The Soviet Model - Epidemiological Transition - Post-Soviet Reform - Future Prospects - Summary - Israel - Origins of the Israeli Health System - Health Resources and Expenditures - Health Reforms - Mental Health - Healthy Israel 2020 - Quality Assurance - Summary - Health Systems in Developing Countries - Federal Republic of Nigeria - Female Genital Mutilation - Communicable Diseases - Non-Communicable Diseases - Nigeria's Health System - Millennium Development Goals - Cancer - HIV/AIDS - Food Fortification/Malnutrition - Health Reform - Summary - Latin America and the Caribbean - Colombia - Asia -

India - China - Japan - Comparing National Health Systems - Economic Issues in National Health Systems - Reforming National Health Systems - Summary - Note - Bibliography - International - United States - Canada - United Kingdom - Europe - Contents note continued: Nordic Countries, Germany, and the Netherlands - Russia - Israel - Developing Countries - Nigeria - Latin America and the Caribbean - Colombia - India - China - Japan - 14.Human Resources for Health - Introduction - Overview of Human Resources - Human Resources Planning - Supply and Demand - Medical Education - Postgraduate Medical Training - Specialization and Family Practice - Training in Preventive Medicine - Nursing Education - In-Service and Continuing Education - Accreditation of Health Professional Educational or Training Facilities - The Range of Health Disciplines - Licensure and Supervision - Constraints on the Health Care Provider - Other Health Professions - Expanding Roles in Primary Care - Nurse Practitioners - Physician Assistants - Feldshers - Community Health Workers - Alternative Medicine - Changing the Balance - Education for Public Health and Health Management - Contents note continued: Core Elements for Master of Public Health Programs - Ranking Universities - Field Epidemiology - Public Health Education in Europe - Health Policy and Management of Human Resources - Summary - Note - Bibliography - 15.Health Technology, Quality, Law, and Ethics - Introduction - Innovation, Regulation, and Quality Control - Appropriate Health Technology - Priority Interventions in Low- and Medium-Income Countries - Priority Selection in High-Income Countries - Health Technology Assessment - Technology Assessment in Hospitals - Technology Assessment in Prevention and Health Promotion - Technology Assessment in National Health Systems - Dissemination of Technology - Diffusion of Technology - Quality Assurance - Adverse Events and Negligence - Licensure and Certification - Health Facility Accreditation - Peer Review - Tracer Conditions - Setting Standards - Algorithms and Clinical Guidelines - Organization of Care - Contents note continued: Diagnosis-

Related Groups - Managed Care - Performance Indicators - Consumerism and Quality - The Public Interest - Total Quality Management - Public Health Law - Environmental Health - Public Health Law Reform - Ethical Issues In Public Health - Individual and Community Rights - Tragic Deviations in Public Health Ethics - Human Experimentation - Ethics in Public Health Research - Ethics in Patient Care - Sanctity of Life Versus Euthanasia - The Imperative to Act or Not Act in Public Health - Summary - Note - Bibliography - Health Technology - Quality - Law - Ethics - 16.Global Health - Introduction - The Global Health Situation - Priorities in Global Health - Poverty-Illness-Population--Environment - Child Health - Maternal Health - Population Growth - Malnutrition - The Fight Against HIV/AIDS and Other Communicable Diseases - Non-Communicable Diseases - Disaster Management - Environment - Contents note continued: Global Partnership for Development - Development and Health - Organization for International Health - World Health Organization - United Nations Children's Fund - Non-Governmental Organizations - The World Bank - Trends in Global Health - Emerging Infectious Disease Threats - Expanding National Health Capacity - Top-Down and Bottom-Up Development - Global Health and the New Public Health - Summary - Note - Bibliography - Global Health - International Organizations - Global Health in the Future. Subjects: Public health. Medical policy. Notes: Previous edition: London: Academic, 2009. Includes bibliographical references and index. Dewey class no.: 362.1

Traumatic childbirth LCCN: 2012050443 Type of material: Book Personal name: Beck, Cheryl Tatano. Main title: Traumatic childbirth / Cheryl Tatano Beck, Jeanne Driscoll, and Sue Watson. Published/Created: Abingdon, Oxon: Routledge, 2013. Description: viii, 255 p.; 24 cm. ISBN: 9780415678094 (hbk.) 9780415678100 (pbk.) LC classification: RG852 .B42 2013 Related names: Driscoll, Jeanne. Watson, Sue, 1958- Summary: "Postpartum depression has become a more recognized mental illness over the past decade as a result of education and increased awareness. Traumatic childbirth, however, is still often overlooked, resulting in a scarcity of information for health professionals. This is in spite of up to 34% of new mothers reporting experiencing a traumatic childbirth and prevalence rates rising for high risk mothers, such as those who experience stillbirth or who had very low birth weight infants. This groundbreaking book brings together an academic, a clinician and a birth trauma activist. Each chapter discusses current research, women's stories, the common themes in the stories and the implications of these for practice, clinical case studies and a clinician's insights and recommendations for care. Topics covered include: mothers' perspectives, fathers' perspectives, the impact on breastfeeding, the impact on subsequent births, PTSD after childbirth and EMDR treatment for PTSD. This book is a valuable resource for health professionals who come into contact with new mothers, providing the most current and accurate information on traumatic childbirth. It also presents mothers' experiences in a manner that is accessible to women, their partners, and families"--Provided by publisher. Contents: What is traumatic birth and posttraumatic stress due to childbirth - Jeanne's introduction to posttraumatic stress disorder secondary to birth trauma - Review of the literature on risk factors for postpartum posttraumatic stress response - Women's narratives of risk factors for posttraumatic stress disorder - Assessment and diagnosis - Case study 1: Carol - Instruments to screen for posttraumatic stress disorder - Impact of traumatic childbirth on breastfeeding - Anniversary of birth trauma - Subsequent childbirth after a previous traumatic birth - Case study 2: Anne - Selected treatments for posttraumatic stress disorder - Case study 3: Sheila - Fathers and traumatic childbirth - Trauma and Birth Stress (TABS) - Secondary traumatic stress. Subjects: Puerperal Disorders--psychology. Stress Disorders, Post-Traumatic. Parturition--psychology. Postnatal Care--psychology. Postpartum Period--psychology. Notes: Includes bibliographical references. Dewey class no.: 618.7/6

Williams manual of pregnancy complications / senior editor, Kenneth J. Leveno; associate editors, James M. Alexander ... [et al.]. Edition: 23rd ed.

Published/Created: New York: McGraw-Hill Professional, c2013. Projected pub date: 1211 Description: p.; cm. ISBN: 9780071765626 (alk. paper) Variant title: Manual of pregnancy compliations Related titles: William's manual of obstetrics. Williams obstetrics. Related names: Leveno, Kenneth J. Alexander, James M., 1965- Summary: "The only pocket manual derived from Williams Obstetrics, 23e - completely updated and now in full color Williams Manual of Pregnancy Complications, 23e is a carry-anywhere, condensed guide to the Williams protocols for diagnosis and management of complications and illnesses during pregnancy. Reflecting the rigorously referenced, evidence-based approach of the parent text, the manual delivers essential information on: Prenatal screening Mediation use in pregnancy Hypertension disorders in pregnancy Pain management dosages Procedures for complicated labor and delivery, hemoglobinopathies, and more Thoroughly cross-referenced to Williams Obstetrics, 23e for the latest literature citations, this edition is enhanced by a new full-color presentation, more tables and algorithms, and an increased emphasis on diagnosis and treatment. There is no faster or more efficient way to access the key facts, diagnostic tools, and treatment guidelines found in Williams Obstetrics, 23e than this authoritative, streamlined sourcebook"--Provided by publisher. Contents: Machine generated contents note: Part I: Obstetrical Complications due to Pregnancy 1. Early Pregnancy Loss 2. Ectopic Pregnancy 3. Screening for Neural-Tube Defects, Down Syndrome, and Heritable Genetic Diseases 4. Prenatal Diagnosis 5. Chromosomal Abnormalities 6. Single-Gene (Mendelian) Disorders 7. Nonmendelian Disorders 8. Teratology, Medications, and Substance Abuse 9. Ultrasound Imaging Including Doppler Velocimetry 10. Oligohydramnios 11. Hydramnios 12. Antepartum Fetal Testing 13. Intrapartum Fetal Heart Rate Assessment 14. Abnormal Labor and Delivery 15. Chorioamnionitis 16. Shoulder Dystocia 17. Breech Delivery 18. Prior Cesarean Delivery 19. Uterine Rupture 20. Hysterectomy Following Delivery 21. Postpartum and Postoperative Infections 22. Septic Pelvic Thrombophlebitis 23. Gestational Hypertension and Preeclampsia 24. Eclampsia

Complications in the Fetus or Newborn Infant 89. Resuscitation of the Newborn Infant 90. Neonatal Complications of Prematurity 91. Rh Disease and Other Isoimmunization 92. Injuries to the Fetus and Newborn 93. Meconium Aspiration, Cerebral Palsy, and Other Diseases of the Fetus and Newborn 94. Stillbirth Appendix A: Diagnostic Indices in Pregnancy Appendix B: Ultrasound Reference Tables Appendix C: Radiation Dosimetry Appendix D: Umbilical Cord Blood Gas Analysis Index . Subjects: Pregnancy Complications--Handbooks. Notes: Rev. ed. of: William's manual of obstetrics / Kenneth J. Leveno ... [et al.]. 22nd ed. c2007. Derived from: Williams obstetrics. 23rd ed. / [edited by] F. Gary Cunningham ... [et al.]. c2010. Includes bibliographical references and index. LCCN: 2012026521 Dewey class no.: 618.2

Index

E

F

G

H

I

J

K

L

M

N

O

P

Q

R

S

T

U

V

W

X

Y

Z